Fundamentalist Religious Childhoods and Adult Mental Health and Wellbeing

"Grounded in her own experience of religious fundamentalism, the author makes the key point that 'there is a dearth of professionals who can work ethically and knowledgably with survivors of religious trauma'. This much-needed book offers a wonderful opportunity for those in the caring professions to gain insight into the true toxicity of religious trauma, which has been a much-neglected area of psychological concern."

—Alistair McBeath, *Senior Lecturer, Metanoia Institute, London, UK*

"Dr. Gill Harvey honors the research documenting the benefits of involvement in religious communities while offering a much-needed, more nuanced discussion of the harmful effects on mental health and wellbeing in later life for those born and/or raised within strict fundamentalist religious settings. Drawing from her personal experience, clinical expertise, and research, Dr. Harvey has provided an invaluable resource for clinicians and other professionals working with those who have experienced developmental religious trauma, which is often unrecognized or unacknowledged. I highly recommend this book!"

—Janyne McConnaughey, *Author of* Trauma in the Pews: The Impact on Faith and Spiritual Practices

"This book names what many survivors have lived but couldn't articulate. It's a compassionate, practical resource for clinicians ready to understand the lasting impact of fundamentalist religious childhoods. Adults raised in these environments have been waiting to be seen, heard, and understood. For professionals committed to trauma-informed care, this guide is essential."

—Rebekah Drumsta, *Author of* When Family Hurts: 30 Days to Finding Healing and Clarity

"Dr. Gill Harvey offers a groundbreaking, compassionate exploration of how fundamentalist religious upbringings shape adult wellbeing. Blending rigorous research with lived experience, this work bridges academic insight and therapeutic wisdom. This book is a vital resource for counsellors and mental health professionals seeking to understand and ethically support those navigating the complex legacies of faith, trauma, and healing. I will be recommending it broadly to clients and therapists alike!"

—Mark Gregory Karris, *Author of* Beyond Fairy Tales: A Couples Guide to Finding Clarity, Doing the Work, and Building a Lasting Relationship

"Gill Harvey, based on her own narrative research, has produced an informative book which contributes significantly to the less-acknowledged area of working therapeutically with adults who have experienced a fundamentalist religious upbringing. It is a balanced, informative and practical tome, which offers useful insights to helping practitioners whose clients may struggle to realise and explore the impact of their upbringing."

—Peter Gubi, *Professor of Counselling and Spiritual Accompaniment, University of Chester, Chester, UK*

"Dr. Gill Harvey's book arises out of her doctoral research into the impact of fundamentalist religious childhoods, drawing on her own personal experience and that of others. She also reflects on the integration of spirituality into counselling, and discusses possible vicarious trauma on professionals involved. As a therapist, her contribution to the literature of religious abuse is both relevant and valuable."

—Lynette Harborne, *Author of* Spirituality and Psychotherapy, Two Languages, One Voice?

Gill Harvey

Fundamental ist Religious Childhoods and Adult Mental Health and Wellbeing

palgrave
macmillan

Gill Harvey
Counselling Psychology and Psychotherapy
Metanoia Institute
London, UK

ISBN 978-3-032-20139-3 ISBN 978-3-032-20140-9 (eBook)
https://doi.org/10.1007/978-3-032-20140-9

Cover illustration: ©FatCamera/Getty Images

This Palgrave Macmillan imprint is published by the registered company Springer Nature Switzerland AG
The registered company address is: Gewerbestrasse 11, 6330 Cham, Switzerland

My thanks to all of the co-researchers who openly shared their stories of growing up within a strict religion and who gave so willingly and freely of their time. I am deeply grateful to each one of you.

This book is dedicated to them and all those who have been damaged by religious fundamentalism,whether born into, raised or joined as an adult. It is for those who acknowledge the impact, and those who do not yet recognise the benefits and challenges of their strict religious upbringing. For those seeking to heal from these experiences, may you know grace, love, kindness,and trustworthy people to walk alongside you on your journey of recovery. May we, as survivors, continue to reflect on how aspects of fundamentalist religion continue to live within us.

Competing Interests The author has no competing interests to declare that are relevant to the content of this manuscript.

Ethical Approval Ethical approval to proceed with this research project was gained from Metanoia Institute/Middlesex University. All co-researchers gave their informed consent to participation and for the findings to be disseminated through journal articles, books, and conference talks. Self-chosen participant pseudonyms have been used throughout the project and in this publication. Confidentiality and anonymity are also protected by the removal of any identifying material in collaboration with the individual co-researchers.

Contents

About the Author

Gill Harvey D.Psych; BACP (Senior Accredited); ACC (Accredited). Gill is a therapeutic counsellor/psychotherapist, supervisor, and trainer working mainly in private practice. She is also the group supervision lead for the Hummingbird Cancer Centre in Bicester and a Trustee of an affordable counselling service in Bedfordshire. Gill completed a research doctorate at the Metanoia Institute/Middlesex University, the title of her thesis being: 'Both sides of the coin: Counsellors' stories of the influence of a fundamentalist religious upbringing on mental health and wellbeing in adulthood'. She has published several journal articles on the topic and contributed a chapter, 'The impact of completing a doctorate as an older person in a global pandemic and the steps taken to protect my Mental Health' to the Research Handbook of Academic Mental Health published by Edward Elgar. Gill has spoken at conferences both nationally and internationally. Her specialised interest is in early developmental religious experiences and adult mental health and wellbeing, and the relationship between counselling/psychotherapy and spirituality.

List of Figures

List of Tables

Part I

The introduction

1

Introduction

Historic Introduction

Historically, in the United Kingdom (UK), religious abuse has focused on priests' sexual abuse of children and the injustices of Ireland's Magdalene Laundries. The earliest writing about spiritual abuse within the Judeo-Christian tradition originated in the United States of America (USA) (Johnson & Van Vonderen, 1991) and was written for leaders and victims. In the UK, literature started to emerge with the seminal work of Oakley and Kinmond (2013); Oakley and Humphreys (2019), which also focused on Christian churches and organisations, reinforcing the belief that it only occurs there (Swindle, 2017) rather than in strict religious homes and other religions. In recent years, the increased awareness of abuse has generally facilitated growing knowledge about religious trauma, including abuse from religious leaders and towards them. *Adult congregants, older people, teenagers, and children can all be victims and abusers, with the term child abuse linked to faith or belief (CALFB) being adopted for minors.*

Many memoirs of growing up within fundamentalist religious families and groups have been published in recent years. Stott (2017) gives her account of growing up in a high-demand religious sect, while Feldman

G. Harvey, *Fundamentalist Religious Childhoods and Adult Mental Health and Wellbeing*, https://doi.org/10.1007/978-3-032-20140-9_1

(2012) shares her story of a childhood spent in the strictly religious Satmar sect of Hasidic Judaism. Phelps-Roper (2019) writes about being raised in the Westboro Baptist Church, while Westover (2018) provides a moving account of growing up without education or medical intervention, preparing for the end of the world. Selbie (2024) published a combined memoir and survival handbook, having been a Christian minister's wife for many years, but is now a therapist who helps clients deconstruct their relationship with religion.

In the UK, public awareness has also been raised by the report of the independent inquiry into child sexual abuse (IICSA) (2022), which examined how organisations, including religious groups, have exploited children. The Makin review (2024) investigated allegations of the Church of England's failure to effectively process reports of the late John Smyth's prolific abuse of young men. Numerous safeguarding concerns were raised in 2019 about Mike Pilavachi, the founder of Soul Survivor, an evangelical, charismatic Christian organisation, regarding his behaviour with young people. The leaders of the now disbanded Jesus Fellowship have had many allegations of sexual, physical, emotional, and financial abuse, with a victims' redress scheme in place and a television documentary about the group being broadcast in the UK during 2025.

The experiences of young people growing up in strict religious environments and the impact on adult health have been largely neglected, with accounts focusing solely on the traumatic parts. This book considers 'both sides of the coin' in acknowledging that some elements of a strict religious upbringing can be beneficial for some. It is research-based, and even though the benefits of such a childhood come first, the author is most definitely not an apologist but a survivor and professional who works with those who have similar experiences.

Young people can suffer from indisputable harm in their formative years, from fundamentalist religious parents, leaders, and other adults. The impact on adult wellbeing for some adds to the injustice of what they suffered at the hands of those who should have been trustworthy and protected them. To concentrate on just one side of the coin creates an imbalanced and incomplete picture and adds to the injustice. This book aims to give a more rounded picture of some young people's experience than some of the other literature on religious trauma/spiritual abuse.

My Story

My journey, from the strict religious environment that I grew up with, to my life now as wife, mother, grandmother, psychotherapist, supervisor, researcher, writer, and trainer, has taken a long time. It has involved years of therapy and study, including training to be a counsellor and working with many clients over the years, to objectively recognise the toxicity of the dogmatic and legalistic Christianity that my family-of-origin was steeped in. It seems pertinent, however, to return to the start of my story so that the reader can understand the context of my young life.

My early life was spent in the heart of Wales, back in the mid-1950s, where I was born into a working-class, nuclear family which was multi-generationally steeped in chapel religiosity dating back to the Welsh Revival (1904–1905).[1] My early years are recalled as secure, which is not surprising, given the safety of a small, remote town in that era. This sociocultural heritage remained intact until my mother was 'love-bombed'[2] (Singer, 2003, p. 114) and radically converted to an evangelical, high-demand, one-off, now long-defunct, group, which came to the town when I was three years old. Over time, her conversion dramatically altered her parenting style because her faith was based on a literal interpretation of the Bible, resulting in legalism, dogmatism, and strict rules that permeated all aspects of life. The full effects of my mother's conversion became more apparent after the birth of my sister when I was nine years old, and I now believe that she suffered from undiagnosed post-natal depression. The pressure to behave in strictly prescribed ways was real, so I chose to be a good and helpful girl, which gained approval rather than parental anger. Despite this compliance, humiliation and shame were common occurrences while my father failed to protect me from such assaults. My mother became a strict,

[1] The Welsh Revival started in Ebenezer Baptist Church, Abertillery in 1904 with 1,000 people present and spread throughout Wales, and in just over a year more than 100,000 people are thought to have made a commitment to Jesus Christ.

[2] The phrase 'love-bombing' (Singer, 2003, p. 114) refers to the situation where members of a group focus on potential members in a way that showers them with love and importance, thus meeting some basic human needs and further drawing them into the community.

absolutist, authoritarian disciplinarian who used religion as a manipulative tool. Threats that I would go to hell for minor misdemeanours were commonplace, alongside scary tales constantly hanging over me, of 'the second coming of Christ' and the risk of being 'left behind' when it happened. Growing up, attendance at the local Mission Hall three times on a Sunday was mandatory, with hat-wearing, long hair, and skirt length well below the knee required, in order not to tempt men, and with outsiders regarded as 'worldly' (Stott, 2017, p. 18), while we were special as we had the truth.

During those growing-up years, I was confused because while I was taught that God was loving, He would punish me by consigning me to hell for minor misdemeanours. I lived in constant fear, hyper-aroused and hypervigilant to stay safe, with adrenaline constantly flooding my system. This demonstrates that even if biological parents are physically present, the child's nervous system may still be alert (Gerhardt, 2015). Since childhood, I have wondered about the effects of being raised in this way on wellbeing in later life. Dominant control exerted by strict, unhealthy, obsessive, rule-driven religiosity is concerning, given that caregivers who are aware of their offspring's needs and are adaptable help the healthy neural wiring process of their children's brains (Thompson, 2010). In contrast, my needs were rarely considered, with my sense of self battered. I lacked self-confidence and self-esteem, and held deep shame accompanied by core beliefs of being evil. The indoctrination was so great that I pretended that we were a loving Christian family for many years, although love was always conditional. For many years, I somatised my emotions and built my fragile self-concept around doing and saying the right things. Like my siblings, I left home at a young age, in my case, to work for a missionary society. It was there that I met my husband-to-be, and I resolved that should we have a family, our children would be brought up very differently from the way that I had been.

It was in my twenties that I had my first period of ill health, when I was unwell for eighteen months. At the time, I thought it was due to sleep deprivation and the busy life of a young mum with two small children. However, I developed severe ME/CFS (Myalgic Encephalomyelitis/Chronic Fatigue Syndrome) in my late forties, with severe anxiety and depression because my life was shattered. I had started to have some counselling just before becoming ill, even though I had for many years been resistant to talking about my issues. During the time of being housebound, my counselling continued over the telephone, and I lived for the weekly sessions where I had a space to express how hard life was. While I remain grateful for the support I received then and through therapy since, I am convinced that not one of the counsellors that I have worked with has been able to comprehend the influence of my strict religious upbringing on my health. While this might not be possible, an expression of wanting to understand could have positively affected therapeutic outcomes. Someone with a similar background might have been able to empathetically accept the enormity of my childhood situation, but this was not my experience. It was impossible to find a counsellor or spiritual director who could work ethically and knowledgeably with me, despite my search that lasted for many years, which eventually led to this research project.

More Recent Events

Many decades have passed, and both my parents have died in recent years, but the reverberations of growing up with religious fundamentalism have reverberated in toxic relational dynamics that continue to exist up to the present day. In the interests of my health and safety, I had to step back and protect myself by taking the hugely difficult decision to estrange myself from my family of origin. This was a tumultuous decision that led to an indescribable loneliness at my core (Mohammed, 2019), not least because of the shunning and ostracism that I have been subjected to. This 'state of loss or exile' (Laing, cited in Honeyman, 2017, p. x) creates great sadness alongside feeling freer physically, emotionally, spiritually, and psychologically more than ever before, free to be me, to live my life, and to hold my own beliefs and values. This freedom has enabled the pursuit of this project as an insider-researcher, while holding gratitude for learning about faith from a young age and outrage for the way that religion was used to coercively control. The high price I have paid in terms of my adult physical and mental health is grossly unfair.

Despite the upsurge of interest in the topic of religious abuse and the increasing literature on the positive impact of religion and spirituality on functioning (Aten & Leach, 2009), there is a dearth of professionals who can work ethically and knowledgeably with survivors of religious trauma. Consequently, there needs to be more counsellors, psychotherapists, spiritual directors, ministers, rabbis, imams, pastoral carers, and coaches to be psycho-educated on this topic. Growing up in a fundamentalist religious environment is not a homogeneous experience, and there will be commonalities and disparities in the stories shared. I have worked for many years as a psychotherapist, and latterly specialised in working with survivors, and although now semi-retired, I have developed a continuing professional development (CPD) interactive and experiential three-day online workshop for therapists, so that as more people recognise the impact of their formative strict religious experiences on wellbeing, more professionals will be equipped to work with them.

The Essential Nature of Self-Care

While both the benefits and challenges of a strict religious upbringing are covered in this book, readers are encouraged to look after themselves, especially those who are survivors of religious trauma. Even professionals with similar experiences who may have come a long way in their healing can be triggered and dysregulated by a phrase or terminology that they may not have encountered for decades. It is important to pace the reading of the difficult sections and intersperse them with life-enhancing activities that energise and bring joy.

This chapter has set the scene for some of the historic events that have led to greater recognition of religious abuse in contemporary society. My personal story of a fundamentalist religious childhood and adult health challenges has been shared, while the need for the reader to practise self-care has also been stressed. In the next chapter, the challenges of defining key terms such as religious fundamentalism will be highlighted, and contextual information will be provided on concepts such as religion and health.

References

Aten, J. D., & Leach, M. M. (2009). *Spirituality and the therapeutic process, a comprehensive resource from intake to termination.* American Psychological Association.

Feldman, D. (2012). *Unorthodox. The scandalous rejection of my Hasidic roots.* Simon and Schuster.

Gerhardt, S. (2015). *Why love matter. How affection shapes a baby's brain.* Routledge.

Honeyman, G. (2017). *Eleanor Oliphant is completely fine.* HarperCollins.

Johnson, D., & Van Vonderen, J. (1991). *The subtle power of spiritual abuse.* Bethany House.

Mohammed, Y. (2019). *Unveiled. How Western liberals empower radical Islam.* Free Hearts Free Minds.

Oakley, L., & Humphreys, J. (2019). *Escaping the maze of spiritual abuse. Creating healthy Christian cultures.* Society for Promoting Christian Knowledge.

Oakley, L., & Kinmond, K. (2013). *Breaking the silence on spiritual abuse.* Palgrave MacMillan.

Phelps-Roper, M. (2019). *Unfollow. A journey from hatred to hope, leaving the Westboro Baptist Church.* riverrun.

Selbie, J. (2024). *Divorcing religion. A memoir and survival handbook.* Prominence.

Singer, M. T. (2003). *Cults in our midst: The continuing fight against their hidden menace.* Jossey-Bass.

Stott, R. (2017). *In the days of rain. A daughter, a father, a cult.* 4th Estate.

Swindle, P. J. (2017). *A twisting of the sacred: The lived experience of religious abuse* (PhD thesis, University of North Carolina). https://www.proquest.com/openview/2f8757f55d11975590c5affc36b72169/1?pq-origsite=gscholar&cbl=18750

The Makin Review. (2024). https://www.churchofengland.org/media/press-releases/independent-review-churchs-handling-smyth-case-published

The Report of the Independent Inquiry into Child Sexual Abuse. (2022). https://www.iicsa.org.uk/final-report

Thompson, C. (2010). *Anatomy of the soul. Surprising connections between neuroscience and spiritual practices that can transform your life and relationship.* Tyndale House.

Westover, T. (2018). *Educated.* Hutchinson.

2

Definitional Challenges and Contextual Information

Spirituality and Religion

Although not necessarily religious, spirituality generally refers to deep connections with something bigger (Miller, 2023). In contrast, religion has been defined as:

> An organised system of beliefs, practices, rituals and symbols that can be seen to be designed to (a) facilitate closeness to the sacred or transcendent being (God, high power or ultimate truth/reality) and (b) foster an understanding of one's relationship and responsibility to others living together in a community. (Candy et al., 2012, p. 2)

These terms are commonly combined in the literature as spirituality/religion and used interchangeably. This book will continue this tradition.

G. Harvey, *Fundamentalist Religious Childhoods and Adult Mental Health and Wellbeing*, https://doi.org/10.1007/978-3-032-20140-9_2

The Abrahamic Religions

Islam, Judaism, and Christianity are known as the Abrahamic religions. They are 'a group of monotheistic religions who believe in a covenant between God and humankind' (Collins English Dictionary, 2019). Great diversity exists between and within them, so that they can be best understood as on a continuum from liberal and cultural at one end, to the extremely strict at the other, for example, the ultra-orthodox Haredi Jews.

Religion and Health

Some of the research has shown that religious people enjoy better physical and mental health and life satisfaction (Hackney & Sanders, 2003; Koenig, 2001; Koenig et al., 2012). Religious beliefs, identity, practices, and involvement in religious communities have also been found to positively support wellbeing, with hope, optimism, and life satisfaction resulting in shorter bouts of depression (Koenig, 2007, 2009; Smith et al., 2003). Some texts state that religious involvement can reduce the prevalence of drug and alcohol dependence (Cook et al., 1997), with fewer occurrences of juvenile delinquency (Johnson et al., 2000) and suicide completions (Van Praag, 2009). Koenig et al. (2012) assert that religion can positively benefit physical health, and this viewpoint is strengthened by a meta-analysis of cancer patients that found a significant relationship between the two (Jim et al., 2015). In addition, some quantitative longitudinal studies' results have shown correlations between religious activity and greater longevity (Hood et al., 2018; Larson, 2003). Other findings reveal that religious practices can help some people to cope with illness (Koenig, 2009; Larson, 2003), while one grounded theory study recognised religion as a key factor in healing from bereavement, especially in those who have suffered loss as a result of violence (Johnson & Armour, 2016). Research results have also revealed that spiritual practices can be a coping resource in bereavement through meaning-making and finding comfort and hope during grief (Harvey, 2018). Yet some findings are inconclusive, as demonstrated in research about anxiety, because some results have shown that religious affiliates experience less angst, while others have revealed higher levels for more devoted followers (Koenig et al., 2012; Shrieve-Neiger & Edelstein, 2004).

Other texts highlight the 'compensation or correspondence hypothesis' (Kirkpatrick & Shaver, 1990, p. 321), which seeks to clarify whether early attachment interactions are influential to subsequent religious/spiritual beliefs. The 'compensation' proposition suggests that an image of God as constantly loving, personal, and available opens up the possibility of an available, constant, and secure substitute attachment figure. In contrast, the 'correspondence' hypothesis queries whether an individual's attachment to God is reflective of the child-caregiver relationship. While this suggests some circumstances in which both elements of the hypothesis may be correct, the significance of this theory is that positive relationships with caregivers commonly result in a view of God as loving and nurturing, while the opposite experiences are more commonly associated with an image of God as demanding, strict, and punitive (Beck & McDonald, 2004). This hypothesis is binary in perspective and ignores the fact that the two are not necessarily mutually exclusive because a person could initially experience God in one way and later hold the opposing viewpoint.

The literature as a whole can be criticised for generally having a bias towards a positive impact (Hood et al., 2018), with less attention being given to religious belief having a detrimental impact on self-esteem, depression, and schizophrenia (Watters, 1992, cited in Koenig & Larson, 2001). This strengthens Ellis's declaration (1980, 1988, cited in Koenig & Larson, 2001) that the less religious someone is, the more they are likely to be healthy. Harvey's (2018) research findings that spiritual reappraisal was common in bereavement, backs a growing number of studies that show that religious grappling, doubt, questioning the deity, and conflict with others of the same religion can detrimentally influence grief and health and wellbeing (Ellison et al., 2009; Exline et al., 2000; Hwang et al., 2011; Strawbridge et al., 1998).

The conclusions are confusing because they show that while religion can bring benefits, it can also be detrimental to health, although greater space is given to the former, with more focus on religion and mental health compared to physical wellbeing. The biggest critique, though, is that all of this research has been carried out on mostly adult Christian Western participants (Tiliouine et al., 2009). There is only sparse research that has involved other sociocultural groups (Ahmed & Amer, 2012; Tarakeshwar et al., 2001) or young people.

Religion and Health Within the Abrahamic Religions

Some results indicate that holding Islamic beliefs can be beneficial to health (Abu-Raiya & Pargament, 2010; Hamdan & Oman, 2011), with a questionnaire study involving Algerian participants discovering a moderate correlation between Islamic religiosity and subjective wellbeing, health, and life satisfaction (Tiliouine et al., 2009). An Iranian study of twenty-four Shia Muslim patients with major depressive disorders measured the different effects of group Islamic lifestyle psychoeducative interventions (ILPI), compared to eight sessions of behavioural activation (BA) group therapy (Toghyani et al., 2018), and found that while both treatments yielded similar results, the option which utilised teachings in the Qur'an and Hadith was cost-effectively successful in a non-pharmacological way (Toghyani et al., 2018). These outcomes illustrate the important role that meaning (Gerwood, 2005), a sense of psychological wellbeing (Hawkins et al., 1999), social support (Mir et al., 2015), and confidence in God's (Allah's) help can have in a crisis (Cole, 1999). Other work shows that early religious interventions can be efficacious in the treatment of low mood for Muslim adherents when compared to non-religious treatments (Hook et al., 2010; Mir et al., 2015). Such outcomes are contextually understood within Muslim understandings of health and wellbeing as 'a bounty from Allah', with physical or mental distress being sent to assess patience and reliance on Allah and providing 'spiritual growth and purification' (Ahmed & Amer, 2012, p. 16). Belief about the nature of God is viewed as crucial because if a person's belief system is hopeful and flexible (Pargament et al., 2001) rather than rigid, this can positively impact a depressive illness. The reverse is also true because if a strict punishing perspective is held, this can prevent recovery. Consequently, it is concerning that dogmatic beliefs are central to fundamentalist religion. There is some attention on fundamentalist Islam in the literature, and this may slightly help to correct the imbalance of focus on strict Christianity.

The findings on religion and health are limited for Judaism, too. One reason for this may be the separation from society imposed by many fundamentalist Haredi communities (Rier et al., 2008), with a limited number of Jews being willing to engage in research. The outcomes of one questionnaire-based Canadian study showed that Jewish religiosity and mental health were largely unrelated, despite the findings showing that participants who had a higher level of trust in God suffered less anxiety and depression (Rosmarin et al., 2009). While this is puzzling, there may also be cultural influences present, given that Whiteley et al.'s (2017) qualitative idiographic study of four female ex-members of a Haredi Jewish group revealed that mental illness was seen as a failure, which threatened the security of marriages and was morally challenging. There was also great secrecy surrounding mental illness.

One empirical United States (US) study of 315 participants, which compared the levels of self-stigma in depression between Christians and non-Christians, found that those of an evangelical persuasion were most likely to self-stigmatise such illnesses (McGuire & Pace, 2018), although it needs to be taken into consideration that evangelicalism in the USA is different from its UK presentation. Likewise, a quantitative study of views of depression among Hispanic Pentecostals (Santos & Kalibatseva, 2019) found that the causes of depressive illnesses were seen to be socio-relational rather than biological or spiritual. Yet, a seventeen-year longitudinal study of sixty Mormon undergraduate students revealed no correlation between higher levels of religiosity and psychopathology (Bartz et al., 2010).

The literature discussed up to this point in this chapter has revealed differing outcomes in terms of the positive and negative effects of religion on health, with most of the research being on the effects on mental rather than physical health (Hood et al., 2018) and more focus on the benefits than the detrimental impact. In the next part of the paper, the focus will be narrowed down to consider influential factors on children growing up within a fundamentalist religious environment, keeping in mind the first research question: 'Might a fundamentalist religious upbringing be influential on mental health and wellbeing in adulthood?' To this end, the four universal dimensions of religion, namely, 'believing, bonding, behaving and belonging' (Saroglou, 2011, p. 1320), alternatively conceptualised as 'religious community, religious beliefs, and religious practices' (Hatch, 2015, p. 38), will be used as a structural aid.

There has also been a recognition that religion can negatively impact depression if the conviction is that God is punishing, but has a positive effect if the belief system 'promotes optimism and flexibility' (Pargament et al., 2001). Other research has also demonstrated the beneficial effect of religious practices and beliefs being integrated into treatment for low mood (Mir et al., 2015), with findings showing the efficacy of early religious interventions for Muslim adherents when compared to non-religion-based treatments (Hook et al., 2010; Mir et al., 2015). On the one hand, while such research goes a little way to rectifying the imbalance of focus, such studies are more limited than those focusing on Western Christianity. One reason for the limited research on Judaism and health may be the separation from society imposed by many Haredi communities (Rier et al., 2008), thus limiting the number of Jewish participants. On the other hand, a few studies do exist, such as a questionnaire-based Canadian study which found that Jewish religiosity was mainly unrelated to mental health, yet participants with a higher level of trust in God suffered less anxiety and depression (Rosmarin et al., 2009, p. 97). Within Christianity, an empirical US study which surveyed 315 participants, comparing the levels of self-stigma associated with depressive experiences between Christians and non-Christians, found that the highest levels were present for those of an evangelical persuasion (McGuire & Pace, 2018).

Religious Fundamentalism

The focus of this book is on one form of religious expression within the Abrahamic conventions, namely fundamentalism, a very contentious word. Various definitions exist. Although lengthy and dated, the explanation used most regularly in the psychological literature is:

> … the belief that there is one set of religious teachings that clearly contains the fundamental, basic, intrinsic, essential, inherent truth about humanity and the deity, that this essential truth is fundamentally opposed by forces of evil, which must be vigorously fought; that this truth must be followed today according to the fundamental, unchangeable practices of the past, and that those who believe and follow these fundamental teachings have a special relationship with the deity. (Altemeyer & Hunsberger, 1992, p. 118)

The challenges of delineating religious fundamentalism continue, as there are at least four different questionnaires which seek to measure the extent to which a person believes in fundamentalistic dogma (Hood et al., 2018). These include those devised by Altemeyer and Hunsberger (2004), Fulton et al. (1999), Streib (2008), and Williamson et al. (2010). However, all can be critiqued for their intrinsic reliance on the originator's understanding of the meaning of fundamentalism. One writer suggests that the metaphor of a continuum can be helpful to understanding the differences between 'a flexible, symbolic, and open-minded style versus a rigid, literal, and closed-minded approach to religious interpretation and understanding; the high end of the spectrum reflecting orthodoxy, conservatism, and fundamentalism' (Saroglou, 2021, p. 7). This visual concept aids comprehension of fundamentalism, as do the provided examples, such as the church of Jesus Christ of Latter-day Saints.[1] Jehovah's Witnesses, Islamic fundamentalist groups, Christian Evangelicals, including Pentecostals, the ultra-orthodox Jewish community,[2] and some new religious movements (lannaccone, 1994; Streib et al., 2009). It is crucial to refocus on the differences that exist within and between the Abrahamic conventions and individual groups, some at the fundamentalist, cultic end of the spectrum. Although no globally accepted definition of cults currently exists (Kern & Jungbauer, 2020), the boundary between what is known as a cult and a fundamentalist religious group is blurred.

Barr (1977, pp. 1–2) states that fundamentalist religion is often viewed as 'bad', and there is frequent resistance to the use of it by

[1] The Church of Jesus Christ of Latter-day Saints is also known as the Mormons.

[2] The ultra-orthodox Jewish Community is also referred to as Haredi Jews.

those categorised in this way, particularly within Christianity, because it is regarded as 'a hostile and opprobrious term, suggesting narrowness, bigotry, obscurantism and sectarianism'. Other writers agree with this stigmatisation and negative portrayal (Hood et al., 2005) of it as cognitively rigid (Altemeyer & Hunsberger, 1992, 2004) and prejudiced (Hall et al., 2010; McCleary et al., 2011; Whitley, 2009), which can cause psychological damage (Cornah, 2006, p. 2). What has often been overlooked are the positive effects of certainty, having a sense of purpose and meaning in life, with well-defined rules to follow, which can provide a framework of religious coping strategies (Phillips et al., 2015).

Religious and Spiritual Abuse

The terms 'spiritual abuse' and 'religious abuse' tend to be used interchangeably, and the meaning of such terms has been grappled with at length (Oakley, 2018). Oakley and Kinmond (2013, p. 7) state that '*the impact of limited research into, and understanding of, the experience of spiritual abuse has led to the current position where defining the term spiritual abuse is highly problematic*'. Yet, they give a clear definition of it within Christianity:

> Spiritual abuse is the coercion and control of one individual by another in a spiritual context. The target experiences spiritual abuse as a deeply emotional personal attack. This abuse may include: manipulation and exploitation, enforced accountability, censorship of decision-making, requirements for secrecy and silence, pressure to conform, misuse of scripture or the pulpit to control behaviour, requirement of obedience to the abuser, the suggestion that the abuser has a 'divine' position and isolation from others, especially those external to the abusive context. (Oakley & Kinmond, 2013, p. 21)

A simpler definition also exists: 'spiritual abuse is the mistreatment of a person who needs help and support or increased spiritual empowerment with the result of weakening, undermining or decreasing the person's spiritual empowerment' (Johnson & Van Vonderen, 1991, p. 20). A crucial realisation is that ministers of religion and spiritual leaders can also be abused, by those in authority over them and by their congregants.

Trauma

The word trauma is frequently used in common parlance and has become a buzzword in the counselling and psychotherapy profession in recent years, and yet, like many of the terms in this chapter, explaining it is not straightforward. Definitions range from 'trauma is anything that injures the self – the heart and the soul' (Pasquale, 2015, p. 20), 'something that pierces or wounds our psychological defences' (Powell, 2009, p. 42), to 'exposure to actual or threatened death, serious injury or sexual violence in which intense fear, horror or helplessness predominates' (Sanderson, 2013, p. 17).

While 'trauma is a fact of life' (Levine, 2010, p. xiii), conceptual understanding of it appears to be diverse. Differentiation is often made between psychological trauma, 'the response of the mind and nervous system to an experience that is so overwhelmingly frightening and life threatening that it cannot come to terms with it' (Rothschild, 2011, p. 18), and physical trauma such as 'an emergency medical condition, including brain damage … that may be caused by a traumatic event' (Rothschild, 2011, p. 18). Traumas are often categorised as 'big-T' life-threatening or 'little-t non-life-threatening' (Lee Cori, 2007, p. 2) or 'Type I characterised by a single traumatic event and Type II involving multiple, prolonged and repeated trauma' (Sanderson, 2020, p. 21). It is important to reiterate that although trauma is not always caused by abuse, it includes:

> … any experience that overwhelms a person's ability to cope and often is combined with a sense of helplessness, fear, and horror at what has happened … Trauma, in some ways, is defined by the person experiencing it. Trauma, then, is an overarching concept and refers to any event that is negative, overwhelming, and has significant implications for a person's future. (Levers, 2023, pp. 429–430)

Similarly, psychological trauma can be defined as 'a deeply distressing or disturbing experience' often involving 'emotional shock following a stressful event or physical injury, which may lead to long-term neurosis' (Oxford Living Dictionary, 2019). This definition encompasses a wide range of human experiences from life events such as divorce or bereavement to more extreme events, including involvement in war, being displaced, or raped. While some believe that life-threatening events which exceed a person's normal coping resources are the most traumatic, it is the effect on that person rather than the actual incident that is most crucial. For example, two people might experience the same event, such as being burgled in very different ways, but will have different levels of resilience and abilities to bounce back from and process traumatic incidents. There is even 'considerable variation in what is meant by trauma amongst clinicians, researchers, practitioners and survivors' (Sanderson, 2013, p. 17), with the Diagnostic and Statistical Manual of Mental Disorders (DSM-5) listing of trauma-related disorders being criticised for being too narrow. Yet, in recent years, the DSM criteria for post-traumatic stress disorder (PTSD) were broadened to include 'the witnessing of such traumatic events or learning about such events happening to a close family member or friend' (Sanderson, 2013, p. 18).

Trauma affects each person differently, with some people being hardly impacted at all, while for others it 'is a kind of shattering' (McBride, 2025, loc. 326). DSM-5 combines trauma with stress-related disorders and reiterates that 'psychological distress following exposure to a stressful event is quite variable' (American Psychiatric Association, 2013, p. 265). This leads to the development of PTSD, complex post-traumatic stress disorder (C-PTSD), or dissociative identity disorder (DID) for some. However, it is important to note that not all trauma leads to the development of DID (multiple personalities), PTSD (Shalev & Yehuda, 1998, cited in Tehrani, 2004), or C-PTSD.

McConnaughey (2022, p. 9) describes PTSD as 'a psychiatric disorder that may develop when an individual experiences or witnesses a traumatic, often life-threatening event'. She argues that 'both learning and biological factors' can contribute to the development of PTSD, with survivors being triggered by events in the here and now which remind them of the traumatic experience(s). McConnaughey (2022,

p. 19) also states that the body responds by flooding itself with 'stress hormones', and that the prefrontal cortex temporarily shuts down, as if the traumatic event is happening again. 'Flashbacks are frightening experiences commonly reported by traumatised individuals' (Cozolino, 2010, p. 274). Such experiences can evoke intensely frightening thoughts and memories, causing victims to live with heightened emotions such as anxiety and panic, and remain on high alert for any danger to their survival. McChesney (2025, pp. 21–22) states that PTSD can develop after a single traumatic incident or through the cumulative effects of multiple events, and notes that PTSD 'causes complex, sometimes rapid, and unexpected changes to consciousness'. He criticises the overuse of terms such as trauma and PTSD but also makes a helpful distinction between moral injury—'more values- or conscience-based'—and PTSD—'more fear- or threat-based'. Conversely, McConnaughey (2022, p. 15) argues that while C-PTSD is not listed in DSM-5, it is recognised by many mental health professionals as arising from 'long-term exposure to traumatic stress or repeated traumatic events that have typically occurred in childhood'. Karris (2023, p. 6) further states that C-PTSD is believed to originate from abuse or neglect in childhood, followed by later trauma/s. The three categories of symptoms are 're-experiencing the traumatic event through intrusive memories, nightmares or flashbacks; avoiding experiences relating to the trauma; and feeling hypervigilant as a default state where one's nervous system is on alert, expecting peril at any moment'. He additionally posits that the results of religious trauma can be C-PTSD, given that the condition is a common outcome of longer-term relational situations (sometimes known as betrayal trauma) rather than one-off events. This is very applicable to the focus of this publication, which is on children and young people who are frequently victims of relational trauma/abuse in their religious community and/or at home.

While the understanding of trauma can be narrow, abuse in all its forms, physical, spiritual, sexual, psychological, and emotional, is usually included. However, 'it is the degree of trauma, the context of trauma, and how we experience and understand our experience of that trauma that are all significant in whether it becomes a neurotic nucleus' (Tudor & Tudor, 2009, p. 138).

Religious Trauma

This has been defined as resulting from:

> …. an event, a series of events, relationships, or circumstances within or connected to religious belief, practices, or structure that is experienced by an individual as overwhelming or disruptive and has lasting adverse effects on a person's physical, mental, social, emotional or spiritual wellbeing. (North American Committee for Religious Trauma, 2020)

Anderson (2023) argues that it is a physiological reaction to an event that happens in a religious setting, while Marich (2024, p. 9) defines trauma as 'any unhealed human wound'. Pertinently, she asserts that power inequity causes abuse to be traumatic. Marich (2024, p. 5) also writes about 'the shitty things' that people can do to each other in the name of religion or spirituality that can wound and detrimentally impact mental health. Her perspective is that religious trauma can happen in 'mainstream churches, houses of worship (and) retreat centres'. She highlights that cult-like dynamics can develop in homes when adults are involved in an abusive system, resulting in the weaponisation of religion and the wounding of vulnerable children who are reliant on their caregivers for survival.

Developmental Religious Trauma

This term is commonly used to describe trauma that is suffered in the formative stage of life (infancy until the early twenties), but it is not listed in the DSM as a specific diagnosis (Pasquale, 2015, p. 61). However, it differs from single-event trauma, which involves exposure to a single traumatic incident; developmental trauma is a term used to conceptualise distress characterised by repeated exposure, often within interpersonal relationships and ongoing (Frogley, 2018; Lanktree et al., 2012). The detrimental effects of long-term exposure to trauma can include complex PTSD symptoms such as intrusive memories, nightmares, and constantly being on alert due to a pervading sense of threat. Other associated symptoms can include relational difficulties, a negative self-concept and struggles to regulate, being common (UK Trauma Council, 2020).

There is a lack of uniformity in diagnostic criteria for trauma between the DSM-5 (American Psychiatric Association, 2013) and the International Classification of Diseases (ICD-11) (World Health Organisation, 2018). Complex PTSD is listed in ICD-11 (WHO, 2018), although not everyone suffering with symptoms suggestive of this condition meets the diagnostic criteria despite functional struggles (Mental Health Today, 2019). Those exposed to trauma, especially in their formative years, often have a range of co-morbid physical and mental health problems, although the link to traumatic events often goes unrecognised (The National Institute for Health Research (NIHR), 2021). Some texts highlight the importance of not assuming that trauma results in damage (Joseph, 2015, p. 5), as post-traumatic growth can occur (Tedeschi & Calhoun, 1995). The debate around the appropriateness and usefulness of diagnostic criteria (Frogley, 2018) is ongoing.

In this research study, 'religion' and 'religious trauma' were used to reflect the narrow religious environments in which most co-researchers grew up. However, the complexity of semantics has become apparent in exploring the meaning of terms such as spirituality, religion, spiritual abuse, and religious trauma. The challenge continues as religious fundamentalism is explored in the next section.

Equality, Diversity, and Inclusion

Researchers must value equality, diversity, and inclusionso that participants are treated in an anti-discriminatory way. In line with this, the National Institute for Clinical Excellence (NICE) guidelines encourage researchers' sensitivity to cultural, ethnic, and religious matters. Hearing the co-researchers' stories and their resultant worldviews with an open mind was an essential but integral part of this study.

While most of the literature concentrates on Christianity, the wider focus was an attempt to gain broader insights. However, as can be seen from the co-researcher profile summaries in Table 2.1, although there was some diversity, it was limited, as the majority of participants grew

Table 2.1 Co-researchers' profile summaries

Chosen pseudonym	Gender	Age range	Race and ethnicity	Self-identified religion of upbringing
Co-researcher 1 Holly	Female	50–59	White British	Christianity: Evangelical Baptist
Co-researcher 2 Francesca Alexandra	Female	50–59	White British	Christianity: Assemblies of God Pentecostal
Co-researcher 3 Hannah	Female	40–49	White British	Judaism: Liberal
Co-researcher 4 Eva	Female	40–49	White British	Christianity: Jehovah's Witnesses
Co-researcher 5 Anna4	Female	50–59	White British	Christianity: Evangelical Baptist
Co-researcher 6 Rupert	Male	70+	White British	Christianity: Evangelical Baptist
Co-researcher 7 Maya	Female	21–29	Pakistani British	Islam: Sunni

up within Christianity, although one grew up in a Sunni Muslim family and another in a liberal, cultural Jewish household.

References

Abu-Raiya, H., & Pargament, K. I. (2010). Empirically based psychology of Islam: Summary and critique of the literature. *Mental Health, Religion & Culture, 14*(2), 93–115. https://doi.org/10.1080/13674670903426482

Ahmed, S., & Amer, M. M. (2012). *Counselling Muslims. Handbook of mental health issues and interventions*. Taylor and Francis.

Altemeyer, B., & Hunsberger, B. (2004). A revised religious fundamentalism scale: The short and sweet of it. *International Journal for the Psychology of Religion, 14*, 47–54. https://doi.org/10.1207/s15327582ijpr1401_4

Altemeyer, B., & Hunsberger, B. (1992). Authoritarianism, religious fundamentalism, quest, and prejudice. *International Journal for the Psychology of Religion, 2*, 113–133. https://doi.org/10.1207/s15327582ijpr0202_5

American Psychiatric Association. (2013). *Diagnostic and statistical manual of mental disorders* (5th ed.). American Psychiatric Association.

Anderson, L. E. (2023). *When religion hurts you. Healing from religious trauma and the impact of high-control religion.* Brazos Press.

Barr, J. (1977). *Fundamentalism.* Wipf and Stock.

Bartz, J. D., Richards, P. S., Smith, T. B., & Fischer, L. (2010). A 17-year longitudinal study of religion and mental health in a Mormon sample. *Mental Health, Religion & Culture, 13*(7–8), 683–695. https://doi.org/10.1080/13674670801944966

Beck, R., & McDonald, A. (2004). Attachment to God: The attachment to God inventory, tests of working model correspondence, and an exploration of faith group differences. *Journal of Psychology and Theology, 32*(2), 92–103. https://doi.org/10.1177/009164710403200202

Candy, B., Jones, L., Varagunam, M., Speck, P., Tookman, A., & King, M. (2012). *Spiritual and religious interventions for wellbeing of adults in the terminal phase of disease* (Cochrane review). http://onlinelibrary.wiley.com/doi/101002/14651858CD007544.pub2/abstract

Cole, B. S. (1999). *The integration of spirituality and psychotherapy for people confronting cancer. An outcome study*. Bowling Green State University.

Collins English Dictionary. (2019). https://www.collinsdictionary.com/dictionary/english/abrahamic

Cook, C. H., Goddard, D., & Westall, R. (1997). Knowledge and experience of drug use amongst church affiliated young people. *Drug Alcohol Dependence, 46*, 9–17. https://doi.org/10.1016/S0376-8716(97)00036-7

Cornah, D. (2006). *The impact of spirituality on mental health.* Mental Health Foundation.

Cozolino, L. (2010). *The neuroscience of psychotherapy. Healing the social brain* (2nd ed.). W. W. Norton.

Ellison, C. G., Burdette, A. M., & Hill, T. D. (2009). Blessed assurance: Religion, anxiety, and tranquillity among US adults. *Social Science Research, 38*(3), 656–667. https://doi.org/10.1016/j.ssresearch.2009.02.002

Exline, J. J., Yali, A. M., & Sanderson, W. C. (2000). Guilt, discord, and alienation: The role of religious strain in depression and suicidality. *Journal of Clinical Psychology, 56*(12), 1481–1496. https://doi.org/10.1002/1097-4679(200012)56:12%3c1481::AID-1%3e3.0.CO;.2-A

Frogley, C. (2018, August 3). *Developmental trauma: How useful is this framework?* Association for Child and Adolescent Mental Health. [Blog] https://www.acamh.org/blog/developmental-trauma-useful-framework/

Fulton, A. S., Gorsuch, R. L., & Maynard, E. A. (1999). Religious orientation, antihomosexual sentiment, and fundamentalism among Christians. *Journal for the Scientific Study of Religion, 38*(1), 14–22. https://doi.org/10.2307/1387580

Gerwood, J. (2005). A case of overcoming substance abuse by finding meaning anchored in a religious experience. *International Forum for Logotherapy, 28*, 38–42.

Hackney, C. H., & Sanders, G. S. (2003). Religiosity and mental health: A meta-analysis of recent studies. *Journal for the Scientific Study of Religion, 42*(1), 43–55. https://doi.org/10.1111/1468-5906.t01-1-00160

Hall, D. L., Matz, D. C., & Wood, W. (2010). Why don't we practice what we preach? A meta-analytic review of religious racism. *Personality and Social Psychology Review, 14*, 126–139. https://doi.org/10.1177/1088868309352179

Hamdan, A., & Oman, D. (2011). *Religiosity, spirituality, and mental health: Review of research with Muslim populations, explanatory mechanisms, and future directions.* Manuscript submitted for publication.

Harvey, G. (2018). The impact of client spirituality when bereavement is the presenting issue. *Thresholds, Counselling with spirit.* April 2018, 15–19.

Hatch, T. G. (2015). *Mishpacha in the America diaspora: An exploratory study of highly-involved Jewish families* (PhD thesis, Louisiana State University). http://digitalcommons.lsu.edu/gradschool_dissertations/519.

Hawkins, R. S., Siang-Yang, T., & Turk, A. A. (1999). Secular versus Christian inpatient cognitive-behavioral therapy programs: Impact on depression and spiritual well-being. *Journal of Psychology and Theology, 27*(4), 309–318. https://doi.org/10.1177/009164719902700043

Hood, R. W. Jr, Hill, P. C., & Spilka, B. (2018). *The psychology of religion: An empirical approach* (5th ed.) Guildford Press.

Hood, R. W., Hill, P. C., & Williamson, W. P. (2005). *The psychology of religious fundamentalism.* Guildford Press.

Hook, J. N., Worthington, E. L., Davis, D. E., Jennings, D. J., Gartner, A. L., & Hook, J. P. (2010). Empirically supported religious and spiritual therapies. *Journal of Clinical Psychology, 66*(1), 46–72. https://doi.org/10.1002/jclp.20626

Hwang, K., Hammer, J. H., & Cragun, R. T. (2011). Extending religion-health research to secular minorities: Issues and concerns. *Journal of Religion and Health, 50*(3), 608–622.
Iannaccone, L. R. (1994). Why strict churches are strong. *American Journal of Sociology, 99*(5), 1180–1211. https://doi.org/10.1086/230409
Jim, H. S. L., Pustejovsky, J. E., Park, C. L., Danhauer, S. C., Sherman, A. C., Fitchett, G., Merluzzi, T. V., Munoz, A. R., George, L., Snyder, M. A., & Salsman, J. M. (2015). *Religion, spirituality, and physical health in cancer patients: A meta-analysis.* wileyonlinelibrary.com. https://doi.org/10.1002/cncr.29353
Johnson, B., Larson, D., & McCullough, M. (2000). A systemic review of the religiosity and delinquency literature: A research note. *Journal of Contemporary Criminal Justice, 16*, 32–52. https://doi.org/10.1177/1043986200016001003
Johnson, D., & Van Vonderen, J. (1991). *The subtle power of spiritual abuse.* Bethany House.
Johnson, S. K., & Armour, M. P. (2016). Finding strength, comfort, and purpose in spirituality after homicide. *Psychology of Religion and Spirituality., 8*(4), 277–288.
Joseph, S. (2015). A person-centred perspective on working with people who have experienced psychological trauma and helping them to move forward to posttraumatic growth. *Person-Centred and Experiential Psychotherapies, 14*(3), 178–190. https://doi.org/10.1080/14779757.2015.1043392
Karris, M. G. (2023). *The diabolical trinity.* SacraSage.
Kern, C., & Jungbauer, J. (2020). Long-term effects of a cult childhood on attachment, intimacy and close relationships: Results of an in-depth interview study. *Clinical Social Work Journal, 2020.* https://doi.org/10.1007/s10615-020-00773-w
Kirkpatrick, L. A., & Shaver, P. R. (1990). Attachment theory and religion: Childhood attachments, religious beliefs, and conversion. *Journal for the Scientific Study of Religion, 29*(3), 315–335. https://doi.org/10.2307/1386461
Koenig, H. G. (2001). Religion and medicine II: Religion, mental health, and related behaviors. *The International Journal of Psychiatry in Medicine, 31*(1), 97–109. https://doi.org/10.2190/BK1B-18TR-X1NN-36GG
Koenig, H. G. (2007). Religion and remission of depression in medical inpatients with heart failure/pulmonary disease. *Journal of Nervous and Mental Disease, 195*, 389–395. https://doi.org/10.1097/NMD.0b013e31802f58e3

Koenig, H. G. (2009). Research on religion, spirituality, and mental health: A review. *The Canadian Journal of Psychiatry, 54*(5), 283–291. https://doi.org/10.1177/070674370905400502

Koenig, H. G., King, D. E., & Carson, V. B. (2012). *Handbook of religion and health* (2nd ed.). Oxford University Press.

Koenig, H. G., & Larson, D. B. (2001). Religion and mental health: Evidence for an association. *International Review of Psychiatry, 13*, 67–78. https://doi.org/10.1080/09540260124661

Lanktree, C. B., Briere, J., Godbout, N., Hodges, M., Chen, K., Trimm, L., Adams, B., Maida, C. A., & Freed, W. (2012). Treating multitraumatized, socially marginalised children: Result of a naturalistic treatment outcome study. *Journal of Aggression, Maltreatment and Trauma, 21*(8), 813–828. https://doi.org/10.1080/10926771.2012.722588

Larson, D. B. (2003). Spirituality's potential relevance to physical and emotional health: A brief review of quantitative research. *Journal of Psychology and Theology, 31*(1), 37–51. https://doi.org/10.1177/009164710303100104

Lee Cori, J. (2007). *Healing from trauma. A survivor's guide to understanding your symptoms and reclaiming your life.* Marlowe.

Levers, L. L. (2023). *Trauma counseling: Theories and interventions for managing trauma, stress, crisis and disaster* (2nd ed.). Spring Publishing.

Levine, P. A. (2010). *In an unspoken voice: How the body releases trauma and restores goodness.* North Atlantic Books.

Marich, J. (2024). *You lied to me about God.* North Atlantic Books.

McBride, H. L. (2025). *Holy hurt. Understanding spiritual trauma and the process of healing*. Brazos Press.

McChesney, R. W. (2025). *The soul also keeps the score. A trauma-informed companion to the spiritual exercises of St. Ignatius.* Liturgical Press.

McCleary, D. F., Quillivan, C. C., Forster, L. N., & Williams, R. L. (2011). Meta-analysis of correlational relationships between perspectives of truth in religion and major psychological constructs. *Psychology of Religion and Spirituality, 3*, 163–180. https://doi.org/10.1037/a0022208

McConnaughey, J. (2022). *Trauma in the pews. The impact on faith and spiritual practices.* Berry Powell Press.

McGuire, J. M., & Pace, A. C. (2018). Self-stigma of depression in Christians versus the general population. *Mental Health, Religion & Culture, 21*(6), 601–608. https://doi.org/10.1080/13674676.2018.1522623

Mental Health Today. (2019). *PTSD prevalence research fails to recognise the scope of post-traumatic reactions.* https://www.mentalhealthtoday.co.uk/news/young-people/research-highlights-the-prevelance-of-ptsd-in-young-people-yet-fails-to-recognise-the-scope-of-post-traumatic-reactions

Miller, A. C. (2023). *Religious trauma survival guide. Education & recovery tools for survivors and professionals.* Empathy Paradigm.

Mir, G., Meer, S., Cottrell, D., McMillan, D., House, A., & Kanter, J. W. (2015). Adapted behavioural activation for the treatment of depression in Muslims. *Journal of Affective Disorders, 180*, 190–199. https://doi.org/10.1016/j.jad2015.03.060

National Institute for Health Research. (2021). *Mental health problems in complex trauma: The most promising therapies are identified in a new review.* https://doi.org/10.3310/alert_44248

North American Committee For Religious Trauma Research. (2020). *What is religious trauma?* https://www.gcrr.org/religioustrauma

Oakley, L. (2018). *Understanding Spiritual Abuse.* https://www.churchtimes.co.uk/articles/2018/16-february/

Oakley, L., & Kinmond, K. (2013). *Breaking the silence on spiritual abuse.* Palgrave MacMillan.

Oxford Living Dictionary. (2019). https://en.oxforddictionaries.com/definition/trauma

Pargament, K. I., Tarakeshwar, N., Ellison, C. G., & Wulff, K. M. (2001). Religious coping among the religious: The relationships between religious coping and well-being in a national sample of Presbyterian clergy, elders, and members. *Journal for the Scientific Study of Religion, 40*(3), 497–513. https://doi.org/10.1111/0021-8294.00073

Pasquale, T. B. (2015). *Sacred wounds. A path to healing from spiritual trauma.* Chalice Press.

Phillips, R. E., III., & Ano, G. G. (2015). A re-examination of religious fundamentalism: Positive implications for coping. *Mental Health, Religion & Culture, 18*(4), 299–311. https://doi.org/10.1080/13674676.2015.1022521

Powell, T. (2009). *The mental health handbook. A cognitive behavioural approach* (3rd ed.). Speechmark.

Rier, D. A., Schwartzbaum, A., & Heller, C. (2008). Methodological issues in studying an insular, traditional population: A women's health survery among Israeli Haredi (ultra-Orthodox) Jews. *Women & Health, 48*(4), 363–381. https://doi.org/10.1080/03630240802575054

Rosmarin, D. H., Pargament, K. I., & Mahoney, A. (2009). The role of religiousness in anxiety, depression, and happiness in a Jewish community sample: A preliminary investigation. *Mental Health, Religion & Culture, 12*(2), 97–113. https://doi.org/10.1080/13674670802321933

Rothschild, B. (2011). *8 keys to safe trauma recovery: Take-charge strategies to empower your healing*. Norton.

Sanderson, C. (2013). *Counselling skills for working with trauma*. Jessica Kingsley.

Sanderson, C. (2020). *Adverse childhood experiences*. nscience, 26 June 2020. https://www.nscience.uk/product/healing-the-emotional-and-physical-scars-of-adverse-childhood-experiences/

Santos, L. G., & Kalibatseva, Z. (2019). Perceptions of depression about Hispanics with Pentecostal beliefs. *Mental Health, Religion & Culture, 22*(8), 779–793. https://doi.org/10.1080/13674676.2019.1644305

Saroglou, V. (2011). Believing, bonding, behaving, and belonging: The big four religious dimensions and cultural variation. *Journal of Cross-Cultural Psychology, 42*(8), 1320–1340. https://doi.org/10.1177/0022022111412267

Saroglou, V. (2021). *The psychology of religion*. Routledge.

Shrieve-Neiger, A. K., & Edelstein, B. A. (2004). Religion and anxiety: A critical review of the literature. *Clinical Psychology Review, 24*, 379–397. https://doi.org/10.1016/j.cpr.2004.02.003

Smith, T. B., McCullough, M. E., & Poll, J. (2003). Religiousness and depression: Evidence for a main effect and the moderating influence of stressful life events. *Psychological Bulletin, 129*(4), 614–636.

Strawbridge, W. J., Sherma, S. J., Cohen, R. D., Roberts, R. E., & Kaplan, G. A. (1998). Religiosity buffers effect of some stressors on depression but exacerbates others. *The Journals of Gerontology Series b: Psychological Sciences and Social Sciences, 53B*(3), S118–S126. https://doi.org/10.1093/geronb/53B.3.S118

Streib, H. (2008). More spiritual than religious: Changes in the religious field require new approaches. In H. Streib, A. Dinter, & K. Söderblom (Eds.), *Lived religion: Conceptual, empirical, and practical-theological approaches: Essays in honor of Hans-Günter Heimbroell* (pp. 53–67). Brill.

Streib, H., Keller B., & Silver, C. F. (2009), *Deconversion: Qualitative and quantitative results from cross-cultural research in Germany and the United States of America*. Gottingen: Vandenhoeck & Ruprecht.

Tarakeshwar, N., Pargament, K. I., & Mahoney, A. (2001). Initial development of a measure of religious coping among Hindus. *Journal of Community Psychology, 31*(6), 607–728. https://doi.org/10.1002/jcop10071

Tedeschi, R. G., & Calhoun, L. G. (1995). *Trauma and transformation: Growing in the aftermath of suffering*. Sage.

Tehrani, N. (2004). *Workplace trauma*. Routledge.

Tiliouine, H., Cummins, R. A., & Davern, M. (2009). Islamic religiosity, subjective well-being, and health. *Mental Health, Religion & Culture, 12*(1), 55–74. https://doi.org/10.1080/13674670802118099

Toghyani, M., Kajbaf, M. B., & Ghamarani, A. (2018). Adherence to Islamic lifestyle as a cost-effective treatment for depression. *Mental, Health, Religion & Culture, 21*(8), 797–809. https://doi.org/10.1080/13674676.2018.1551342

Tudor, L. E., & Tudor, K. (2009). Person-centred therapy with trauma and Enactment. In D. Mann & V. Cunningham (Eds.), *The past in the present: Therapy enactments and the return of trauma* (pp. 150–168). Routledge.

UK Trauma Council. (2020). *PTSD and complex trauma*. https://www.uktraumacouncil.org/trauma/ptsd-and-complex-ptsd

Van Praag, T. J. (2009). The role of religion in suicide prevention. In D. Wasserman & C. Wasserman (Eds.), *Oxford textbook of suicidology and suicide prevention*. Oxford University Press.

Whitley, B. E. (2009). Religiosity and attitudes towards lesbians and gay men: Aeta-analysis. *International Journal for the Psychology of Religion, 19*, 21–38. https://doi.org/10.1080/10508610802471104

Whiteley, C., Coyle, A., & Gleeson, K. (2017). An idiographic analysis of women's accounts of living with mental health conditions in Haredi Jewish communities. *Mental Health, Religion & Culture, 20*(3), 277–293. https://doi.org/10.1080/13674676.2017.1354820

Williamson, W. P., Hood, R. W., Jr., Ahmad, A., Sadiq, M., & Hill, P. C. (2010). The Intratextual Fundamentalism Scale: Cross-cultural application, validity evidence, and relationship with religious orientation and the Big Five Factor markers. *Mental Health, Religion & Culture, 13*, 721–747. https://doi.org/10.1080/13674670802643047

World Health Organization. (2018). *International classification of diseases* (11th ed.). (ICD-11). World Health Organization.

Part II

The method of inquiry

3

The Research Project

Design and Methodology

The focus of this chapter is on the study design, otherwise known as 'mapping the territory' (Finlay & Evans, 2009, p. 14). The rationale for choosing qualitative inquiry, rather than quantitative, mixed methods, or action research, will be provided. In the interests of transparency, an outline of other methodologies that were considered will be given, together with the justification for the methodological choices. These were the research questions: 'Might a fundamentalist religious upbringing be influential on mental health and wellbeing in adulthood?' and 'What are counsellors' experiences?'.

Philosophical Positioning

The author's philosophical stance is firmly located within a constructionist-interpretivist perspective combined with a relativist ontological position, and this informs my work as a practitioner and researcher (Penny, 2021), based on the conviction that there is not one truth which can be discovered by hypotheses testing, as humans are

G. Harvey, *Fundamentalist Religious Childhoods and Adult Mental Health and Wellbeing*, https://doi.org/10.1007/978-3-032-20140-9_3

'not passive phenomena waiting to be measured' (Langdridge, 2004, p. 252). Rather, there are a variety of understandings in existence, with experiences being formed and processed through words, and a diversity of applied interpretations (Finlay & Evans, 2009). As indicated in my relativist ontological position with a constructionist stance, this enables me to hold the belief that 'perception and cognition are active processes, in which anything "given" is actually a product of processes, of selection and construction' (Hammersley, 2013, p. 35). It is integrated into my philosophical position because it recognises that 'people's perceptions and experiences are socially, culturally, historically, and linguistically produced' (Finlay & Evans, 2009, p. 19), which is a crucial consideration, given the social, cultural, and historic nature of adult recollections of fundamentalist religious upbringings and the storied nature of the lives of human beings. My perspective is that this blends well with an interpretivist position, which emphasises the essential nature of 'draw(ing) upon our human capacity to understand fellow human beings "from the inside"– through empathy, shared experience and culture etc.' (Hammersley, 2013, p. 26).

These personal viewpoints have led to qualitative methodologies where the focus is on language and the 'deep' (Bottery & Wright, 2019, p. 113) investigation of the subjective experience of the phenomenon in question, rather than the 'Newtonian spirit' (Finlay & Evans, 2009, p. 20), realist ontological perspective of the 'broad' (Bottery & Wright, 2019, p. 113) quantitative testing of hypotheses and the use of numbers and statistics, a mixed methods approach, or action research. The emergence of qualitative methodologies in the last five decades was in reaction to the historically dominant thinking that the purpose of research was to provide rigorous, empirical, and evidential outcomes based on quantitative experiments, measurements, and statistical outcomes. Contrastingly, qualitative studies aim to explore in depth, explain, and interpret the lived experiences of participants (Smith, 2015, p. 21) and seek to understand the richness and complexity of subjective experience (Bright, 2013). Additionally, they explore 'the ways in which people create meaning in their lives' (McLeod, 2015, p. 92). In short, qualitative methodologies involve observing, describing, and interpreting the way that people experience, act on, or think about themselves, their experiences, and the world around them (Bazeley & Jackson, 2013). Despite the influential emergence of qualitative research across many areas of social science, it is convincingly argued that there is little general agreement around methodologies and methods between researchers of a qualitative persuasion, apart from their rejection of quantitative ideology, the result being a plethora of different qualitative approaches, all based on differing ontological and epistemological positions (Hammersley, 2013, p. ix). This critique of qualitative inquiry can also be criticised for the assessment being made through a positivist quantitative lens; the counter-argument is that, given the espoused philosophical positioning of the qualitative mindset, the diversity of opinions is unsurprising. Illustrated in these appraisals is a complete failure to engage with the qualitative universe, but instead to approach research from a quantitative positivist frame of reference. However, I concluded that a qualitative approach was the most appropriate way of researching the questions posed for this study: 'Might a fundamentalist religious upbringing be an influential factor on mental health and wellbeing in adulthood? What are counsellors' experiences?' Because of the phenomenological nature of the research topic, investigating such matters through a quantitative, mixed methods, or action research lens would not align with my philosophical positioning. The concerns of qualitative inquiry are to see through the eyes of research contributors; description of context as important; flexibility; lack of structure; and concepts and theory (Bryman, 2008).

Doing Reflexivity: A Collaborative Narrative Approach

In line with the assertion that 'methodological innovation is the order of the day' (Squire et al., 2014, p. vii), the collaborative narrative approach (Arvay, 1998, 2002, 2003) was developed in response to a perceived lack of qualitative methodology which embodied participants' stories, following the originator's discovery of qualitative research while on a counselling psychotherapy doctoral programme (Arvay, 2003). Being tailor-made, it aims to work collaboratively, to pay attention to the power imbalances frequently present within research projects so that voices are heard and represented; it is underpinned by the belief that 'reality is co-constructed, dialogical, relational, contextual and partial' (Arvay, 2003, p. 163). Its core concepts are collaboration and reflexivity, while being relationally centred, the purpose being to 'co-create research environments that are participatory and emancipatory' (Arvay, 2003, p. 163). What is obvious is the appropriateness of these core concepts to the research topic, given that those who have experienced a fundamentalist religious upbringing were commonly silenced in their developmental years and may not even have verbalised their stories as adults. In the following section, these core concepts of the collaborative narrative approach will be examined in further detail.

The first of these is its relation-centred nature, which is notably recognised by Finlay and Evans (2009) because of its focus on the building of a relational process through the co-creation of 'owning oneself, integrity, reflexivity, acceptance, agency, empathic inquiry, mutuality, openness, impact and humility' (Finlay & Evans, 2009, p. 36). These combine with evidence of 'rigour, relevance, resonance and reflexivity' (Finlay & Evans, 2009, p. 59), thus demonstrating an integral robustness. It is of significance that some findings have shown that participants may be more willing to share their stories with an 'insider-researcher' (De Tona, 2006), thus addressing the imbalance of power in relationships within the research environment.

As the name suggests, collaboration is key to this approach, being defined as 'the act of working together to produce a piece of work, especially a book or some research' (Collins English Dictionary, 2020). Collaboration is demonstrated in practice by all being 'co-investigators' (Arvay, 2003, p. 165) throughout a seven-stage process, rather than the traditional participant and researcher. Greater equity is also facilitated by the interview conversations being a two-way process, in that, rather than just the participant sharing their story, both co-researchers contribute elements of their story in relation to the research topic.

Reflexivity is an essential component of this approach. Distinct from reflection, which is commonly understood as thinking about, reflexivity is more ongoing and a longer-term engagement, as illustrated in Arvay's (2003) perspective of its inclusion as essential because it 'scrutinises the researcher's process and examines how power relations are attended to' (Arvay, 2003, p. 164). It can therefore be understood as a form of critical thinking and appraisal of self and others (Lazard & McAvoy, 2017; Squire et al., 2014), involving 'deliberate self-scrutiny' (Hellawell, 2006, p. 483), revealing the 'underlying assumptions on which arguments and stances are built' (Holland, 1999, p. 467), and questioning inherent 'biases, prejudices, and preconceptions' (Guccione & Wellington, 2017, p. 99). The pertinence of reflexivity to this methodology adds rigour, given that it can be understood as a continual process of internal dialogue and 'critical self-evaluation of the researcher's positionality' (Berger, 2015, p. 220). The fact that reflexivity is such an important part of qualitative inquiry might be challenging for some, particularly those new to qualitative research, since it brings back into focus the polarised binary positions of positivist, objective, quantitative, scientific inquiry versus the anti-positivist subjectivity of qualitative understanding (Lazard & McAvoy, 2017) of the lived experiences of human beings. Nonetheless, despite the 'unhelpful division' (Reicher, 2000, p. 2) of these polarised positions which fails to recognise that there are other approaches between these binary poles such as action research and mixed methods approaches, there can be little doubt that the foundational philosophical building blocks of the qualitative, collaborative, narrative approach (Arvay, 1998, 2002, 2003) make it eminently suited for the exploration of the research topic. Moreover, the structure of the seven-stage process in 'setting the stage – a reflexive preliminary interview; the performance; co-constructing the research interview; the transcription process; four collaborative interpretative readings; the interpretative interview, writing the narratives and sharing the story' (Arvay, 2003, p. 184) confronts those who criticise a lack of structure within Narrative Inquiry generally. Although it is criticised for being 'extensive, time-consuming, very personal' (Arvay, 2003, p. 163), and demanding much from all co-researchers involved, it is respectful to the integrity of participants' stories. Maintaining a stance of 'reflexive criticality' (Guccione & Wellington, 2017, p. 94–100) is surely crucial in the practical application of any methodology; however, the resonances of my fundamentalist religious upbringing mean that this criticality can be challenging for me. Yet,

I hold constant awareness of the importance of criticality as this maintains an attitude of doctorateness and avoids 'methodolatory' (Reicher, 2000; Wellington, 2013).

Study Aims

As previously stated, the methodology was chosen for reasons beyond its current popularity within the social sciences (Squire et al., 2014, p. 1), but mainly because it would facilitate deep exploration of the co-researchers' stories, and meet the aims:

1. to enable co-researchers to tell their own and/or clients' stories on the research topic;
2. to psycho-educate professionals to recognise and understand the influence of a fundamentalist religious upbringing on mental health and wellbeing in adulthood;
3. to add to the sparse literature on this largely hidden topic.

The development of these aims was a crucial undertaking in the early stages of the project, as they enabled me to hold awareness of impact right from the start, thus helping to ensure that the work will 'not remain unread by anyone else beyond my supervisors and examiners' (Dunleavy, 2015, p. 13). The goal for this work is for it to be a 'scholarly contribution' (Dunleavy, 2015, p. 9) that impacts at the macro-level of the counselling and psychotherapy profession and other related caring occupations, but also at the micro-level of interactions between practitioners and clients.

In common with other qualitative work, researcher reflexivity using a written journal was an imperative part of the seven-stage process, as it provided not only a space for personal reflection but also enabled me to stay grounded in my foundational philosophical positioning, the objectives, and ethical considerations. 'Critical reflexivity' (Guccione & Wellington, 2017), involving critical thinking and 'critical being … in the three domains: knowledge, self, and the world' (Barnett, 1997, p. 7) and encompassing self-criticality of my own thoughts, beliefs, faith, and

Table 3.1 The seven-stage process of the collaborative narrative approach (Arvay, 2003)

Stage number	Title
One	Setting the stage
Two	The performance
Three	The transcription process
Four	Four collaborative interpretations of the transcripts
Five	The interpretative interview – a collaborative interpretation of the text
Six	Writing stories
Seven	Sharing the story

knowledge (Guccione & Wellington, 2017, p. 99), has been essential. A summary chart of the seven-stage process is shown in Table 3.1, with the following sections of this chapter exploring each one in greater depth.

Stage One: Setting the Stage

At an early stage, I proposed that up to six co-researchers would be recruited and that they would meet the following criteria:

1. to be qualified counsellors
2. to have grown up in a fundamentalist religious environment within an Abrahamic faith and/or to have worked with clients who had comparable childhoods
3. to have the capacity to provide written informed consent to participate in the research project

Co-researchers were recruited via professional bodies and the counselling training organisation with which I am affiliated, the rationale being that recruitment through such gatekeepers would hopefully aid diversity and access participants who might have been reluctant to volunteer to an unknown sole researcher. The letter of invitation/recruitment poster was emailed to contacts and placed in the research sections of the websites of professional bodies. Anyone interested in possible participation was invited to get in touch so that an information sheet could be forwarded to them.

At that point, the high level of interest in possible participation became clear, as almost fifty enquiries were initially received. The initial conversations took place either online or by telephone, and were structured using a standard form compiled for the purpose, the aim being to build rapport, to start a conversation on the research topic, to explain the commitment involved, and to outline the basic foundational, philosophical positions of the study, especially around the storied nature of our lives (Arvay, 2003). The priority in this phase was 'to facilitate contemplation about the research process' (Arvay, 2003, p. 164) and gauge whether the interested person had the motivation, commitment, and drive for this demanding research method (Arvay, 2003, p. 165). It also gave the opportunity for questions to be asked, and for a pseudonym to be agreed so that in the event of participation, confidentiality and anonymity were protected. A substantial number of interested individuals remained, so 'purposive sampling' (Langdridge, 2007, p. 58; Sandelowski, 1995, p. 180) was used to gain as much diversity of representation as possible, with those not invited to proceed being advised by email. In the interests of procedural transparency, an audit trail of this stage was kept.

Once those invited to continue had accepted, written consent to participate was required, and this included agreeing to the use of their story in the emergent products.

Stage Two: The Performance

During the second stage, the focus moved from recruitment to the building of collaborative relationships and to the one-to-one interviews. Because it is regarded as good practice to offer a choice of interview location (King & Horrocks, 2010, p. 43), co-researchers were asked to indicate their preference regarding the venue from the options of a neutral space, my counselling space, their counselling room, home, or online, the main criteria being 'comfort and quiet' (King & Horrocks,

2010, p. 43). All participants chose to meet in person, with five co-researchers selecting private spaces in their homes, one in her counselling space, and the remainder neutral places. As these interview conversations took place all over the UK during three months, I travelled all over the country. My belief is that the in-person environment in this early phase of the project facilitated the storytelling. This was important, given that the requesting of stories could have been more complex, especially in those early unstructured conversations. All interviews started naturally, with me restating the research questions or through the use of a more general invitation such as 'Tell me about your experiences relating to the research topic' (Atkinson, 1998, p. 29). Despite various 'I' positions being juggled, while conversing in both experiential and reflexive ways (Arvay, 2003), participants generally embodied their stories, and this included recognising 'bodily empathy' and 'embodied intersubjectivity' (Etherington, 2004; Finlay, 2016). This empathy-based approach in the reflexive, collaborative, relational-centred, phenomenological, non-directive, and non-judgemental environment was used as an 'observational strategy' (Stiles, 1993, p. 595), and this aided the attunement. Consequently, some of the inherent power imbalances present in many research interviews were reduced, enabling 'authentic dialogue' (Arvay, 2003, p. 166). The validity and reliability of the storytelling was assisted by inviting co-researchers to begin to tell their stories first, as this avoided any unintentional influence of my own disclosures at the start of conversations. The ability to share elements of my own story in the research interviews was a useful reminder that my contextual role was that of co-researcher. At the end of each stage two interview, each co-researcher was given a debriefing sheet and reminded to make some written reflections if useful.

Stage Three: The Transcription Process

As set out in the Learning Agreement, my original plan was to self-transcribe the interview recordings, as it was my belief that this would enable immersion in the stories and avoid traumatisation of an external transcriber in line with my ethical responsibility 'to do no harm' (Etherington, 2007, p. 85) to an involved party who may have found it difficult to access support (Kiyimba & O'Reilly, 2015, p. 92). Encouraged by one Academic Consultant (AC) to not simply follow prescribed rules, but to engage my 'critical reflexivity' (Guccione & Wellington, 2017), I considered this in the light of the content of stories shared and concluded that traumatisation to a third party was unlikely, whereas a considerable amount of time would be saved. I also decided that immersion in the data was possible without self-transcription. I critiqued Arvay's (2003) insistence that each interview recording be transcribed twice, firstly in rough draft and then in stanza format like a group of lines in a poem, as not only was this pointless but contrary to the collaborative nature of this methodological approach, especially as the plan was to jointly check transcripts with any amendments being agreed between us. Therefore, the decision was taken to utilise the services of an external transcriber.

Stage Four: Four Collaborative Interpretations of the Transcript

This spirit of co-operation continued into the fourth phase as 'the co-investigators and I collaboratively participate(d) to engage the transcribed text in a meaningful way' (Arvay, 2003, p. 169). We individually engaged in four interpretative readings, i.e. reading for content, reading for the self of the narrator, reading for the research question, and reading for relations of power and culture of the transcript. As the complexity of undertaking the four readings of the text became apparent, a reading/interpretative guide was compiled from the information provided and emailed to all participants. Some confusion remained, and therefore an extra online or telephone conversation was arranged with each co-researcher, and this allowed the process to be explained, accompanied by reassurance of my availability to answer questions, should that be necessary. Printed A3 versions of each transcript page were composed, with the interview wording on the left and four columns (one for each interpretative reading) on the right. These forms were then posted to co-researchers, accompanied by four different-coloured pens, one for each interpretative reading. This separate engagement with the transcripts enabled both co-researchers to engage individually in self-reflexivity and criticality, in terms of the interview dynamics and stories shared.

Stage Five: The Interpretative Interview—A Collaborative Interpretation of the Text

In accordance with the collaborative, relational-centred, reflexive spirit of this methodology, a discussion of the four interpretative readings took place between individual co-researchers and me. However, partway through the face-to-face interviews, COVID-19 detrimentally impacted travel, and so, in the interests of safety, the decision was taken to hold the remaining interpretative interviews online. Although the interpretative interviews were complex, the interactions of the 'dialogical construction' (Arvay, 2003, p. 171) were facilitated by our having met each other before, and the conversations were 'very moving and informative' (Arvay, 2003, p. 171). Each conversation was recorded, transcribed, and then checked for accuracy by me only, as in consultation with one of my Academic Consultants, it was felt that if I asked co-researchers to participate in this latter task, there was danger of higher dropp out, given all they had contributed by that stage.

Stage Six: Writing the Stories

By stage six of the process, an enormous amount of storied data had emerged, and the next challenge was to produce a 'pen portrait' (Hollway & Jefferson, 2000, p. 70) for each participant. These portraits served as a 'substitute whole' (Hollway & Jefferson, 2000, p. 70) summary, and allowed stories to be kept intact rather than broken into themes or codes. 'Critical reflexivity' (Guccione & Wellington, 2017) facilitated evaluation of the suggestion that such blended texts needed to be written in the first person to 'bring stories back to life' and avoid objectification (Arvay, 2003, pp. 171–172). The counter-argument was that the stories were already alive, with depictions of narratives written in the third person. This was a pointless exercise and was rejected, together with the suggestion that, due to its time-consuming nature, this stage could be completed without co-researcher input (Arvay, 2003, p. 172). This latter point was counter-intuitive to the collaborative nature of the whole project, especially as it was acknowledged that such a shortcut would compromise the interpretative process (Arvay, 2003, p. 172). Instead, the emphasis continued to be on reflexive, relational-centred collaboration, because this was gauged to be truer to the spirit of the methodology, and consequently, once completed, each 'pen portrait' (Hollway & Jefferson, 2000, p. 70) was sent to the appropriate participant for checking and amendment if necessary. At this point, some participants asked for the removal of material that risked them being identified, and these requests were granted.

Stage Seven: Sharing the Stories

At this point, my focus was on the sharing of stories through the mainly online conferences attended during the COVID-19 era, and the writing of journal articles. The utilised methods were both complex and time-consuming, and yet were respectful to the stories told by each co-researcher of their own and clients' experiences on the research topic. All participants, including the counsellor who withdrew, generously donated their time and efforts.

The Strengths and Weaknesses of the Methods Employed by the Collaborative Narrative Approach

One strength of the collaborative narrative approach (Arvay, 1998, 2002, 2003) is the seven-stage process itself, as it provides a clear structure for the work. This addresses a key critique of Narrative Inquiry that it lacks structure, and yet such a laid-out process might also be perceived as being too prescriptive. Its fundamental constructs of being collaboratively relational-centred and reflexive can be viewed as strengths; yet, given that the focus and aims of the project are decided on before participant recruitment, some inconsistencies are present. This is despite the originator's invitation to make the first steps 'more participatory and emancipatory' (Arvay, 2003, p. 164), which were unachievable for practical reasons, such as the gaining of ethical approval. Guidance around the optimal number of participants when utilising this methodological approach is also lacking, but this is reflective of the wider debate around what might constitute an appropriate sample size for qualitative research. Some argue that this is a much-neglected topic which demands urgent attention (Curtis et al., 2000, p. 102), the greater focus being on data collection and analysis. Others maintain that it is the quality of material obtained 'per sampling unit' (Sandelowski, 1995, p. 179), rather than the number of participants, that is significant. Further debate surrounds the importance of the ontological and epistemological foundations and chosen methodology in determining the number of participants needed (Sim et al., 2018a, 2018b), with some researchers maintaining that it is the extent and nature of the subject matter, the study design, and the attributes of the data (Morse, 2000, p. 3) that count. Helpful indicators include the statement that six to eight participants are normally recommended on UK clinical psychology programmes (Turpin et al., 1997). Langdridge (2007) proposes that a sample of six or fewer participants is appropriate, although this needs to be supported by a balance between methodological requirements and practical feasibility. This observation is backed by Smith (2015), who affirms that sample sizes remaining low enable in-depth exploration and avoid the overwhelm of data. Nonetheless, the debate continues, particularly between those of a quantitative persuasion and those who research the phenomenological experiences of participants.

References

Arvay, M. J. (1998). *Secondary traumatic stress: Stories of struggle and hope* (PhD dissertation). University of Victoria, Canada.

Arvay, M. J. (2002). Putting the heart back into human science research. In J. D. Raskin & S. K. Bridges (Eds.), *Studies in meaning: Exploring constructivist psychology.* Pace University Press.

Arvay, M. J. (2003). Doing reflexivity: A collaborative narrative approach. In L. Finlay & B. Gough (Eds.), *Reflexivity. A practical guide for researchers in health and social sciences* (pp.163–175). Blackwell Science.

Atkinson, R. (1998). *The life story interview.* Sage.

Barnett, R. (1997). *Higher education: A critical business.* SRHE/Open University Press.

Bazeley, P., & Jackson, K. (2013). *Qualitative data analysis: Practical strategies.* Sage.

Berger, R. (2015). Now I see it, now I don't: Researcher's position and reflexivity in qualitative research. *Qualitative Research, 15*(2), 219–234. https://doi.org/10.1177/1468794112468475

Bottery, M. & Wright, N. (2019). *Writing a watertight thesis: A guide to successful structure and defence.* Bloomsbury Academic.

Bright, G. (2013). Making sense of 'ologies.' In G. Bright & G. Harrison (Eds.), *Understanding research in counselling* (pp. 55–94). Sage.

Bryman, A. (2008). *Social research methods* (3rd ed.). Oxford University Press.

Collins English Dictionary. (2020). https://www.collinsdictionary.com/dictionary/collaboration.

Curtis, S., Gesler, W., Smith, G., & Washbourn, S. (2000). Approaches to sampling and case selection in qualitative research: Examples in the geography of health. *Social Science & Medicine, 50*, 1001–1014. https://doi.org/10.1016/S0277-

De Tona, C. (2006). But what is interesting is the story of why and how migration happened. *Forum: Qualitative Social Research, 7*(13). https://doi.org/10.17169/fqs-7.3.143

Dunleavy, P. (2015). *Authoring a PHD. How to plan, draft, write and finish a doctoral thesis or dissertation.* Palgrave.

Etherington, K. (2004). *Becoming a reflexive researcher: Using our selves in research.* Jessica Kingsley.

Etherington, K. (2007). Working with traumatic stories: From transcriber to witness. *International Journal of Social Research Methodology, 10*(2), 85–97. https://doi.org/10.1080/13645570701334001

Finlay, L. (2016). Being a therapist-researcher doing relational-reflexive research. *The Psychotherapist, 62*, 6–7.

Finlay, L., & Evans, K. (2009). *Relational-centred research for psychotherapists.* Wiley.

Guccione, K., & Wellington, J. (2017). *Taking control of writing your thesis.* Bloomsbury Academic.

Hammersley, M. (2013). *What is qualitative research?* Bloomsbury Academic.

Hellawell, D. (2006). Inside-out: Analysis of the insider-outsider concept as a heuristic device to develop reflexivity in students doing qualitative research. *Teaching in Higher Education, 11*(4), 384–494. https://doi.org/10.1080/13562510600874292

Holland, R. (1999). Reflexivity. *Human Relations, 52*(4), 463–484.

Hollway, W., & Jefferson, T. (2000). *Doing qualitative research differently. Free association, narrative, and the interview method.* Sage.

King, N., & Horrocks, C. (2010). *Interviews in qualitative research.* Sage.

Kiyimba, N., & O'Reilly, M. (2015). An exploration of the possibility for secondary traumatic stress among transcriptionists: A grounded theory approach. *Qualitative Research in Psychology, 13*(1), 92–108. https://doi.org/10.1080/14780887.2015.1106630

Langdridge, D. (2004). *Research methods and data analysis in psychology.* Pearson Education.

Langdridge, D. (2007). *Phenomenological psychology: Theory, research and method.* Pearson Prentice-Hall.

Lazard, L., & McAvoy, J. (2017). Doing reflexivity in psychological research: What's the point? What's the practice? *Qualitative Research in Psychology, 17*(2), 159–177. https://doi.org/10.1080/14780887.2017.1400144

McLeod, J. (2015). *Doing counselling research* (3rd ed.). Sage.

Morse, J. M. (2000). Determining sample size. *Qualitative Health Research, 10*(1), 3–5.

Penny, J. E. (2021). The 'research pond'; underlying assumptions in research. *Waverley Abbey College Journal, 1*(1). https://doi.org/10.52456/WACJ0112

Reicher, S. (2000). Against methodolatry: Some comments on Elliott, Fischer, and Rennie. *British Journal of Clinical Psychology, 39*, 1–6. https://doi.org/10.1348/014466500163031

Sandelowski, M. (1995). Sample size in qualitative research. *Research in Nursing and Health, 18*, 179–183. https://doi.org/10.1002/nur.4770180211

Sim, J., Saunders, B., Waterfield, J., & Kingstone, T. (2018a). The sample size debate: Response to Normal Blaikie. *International Journal of Social Research Methodology, 21*(5), 643–646. https://doi.org/10.1080/13645579.2018.1454642

Sim, J., Saunders, B., Waterfield, J., & Kingstone, T. (2018b). Can sample size in qualitative research be determined a priori? *International Journal of Social Research Methodology, 21*(5), 619–634. https://doi.org/10.1080/13645579.2018.1454643

Smith, J. A. (2015). *Qualitative psychology, A practical guide to research methods* (3rd ed.). Sage.

Squire, C., Davis, M., Esin, C., Andrews, M., Harrison, B., Hyden, L.-C., & Hyden, M. (2014). *What is narrative research?* Bloomsbury Academic.

Stiles, W. B. (1993). Quality control in qualitative research. *Clinical Psychology Review, 13*, 593–618. https://doi.org/10.1016/0272-7358(93)90048-Q

Turpin, G., Barley, V., Beail, N., Scaife, J., Slade, P., Smith, J. A., & Walsh, S. (1997). Standards for research projects and theses involving qualitative methods: Suggested guidelines for trainees and courses. *Clinical Psychology Forum, 108*, 3–7.

Wellington, J. (2013). Searching for 'doctorateness.' *Studies in Higher Education, 38*(10), 1490–1503.

4

A Sense of Belonging That Can Be Found Within Religious Families and Communities

Bonding and Belonging in Fundamentalist Religious Families

The form of religion a family subscribes to may be significantly influential on closeness, as seen with Rupert, who felt secure in his growing-up years.

> *… the love in the family was definite. I count myself fortunate that it was from grandparents, parents, and the church.*

Some literature suggests that early infant bonding with a primary caregiver is crucial to health in later life (Aguado, 2018), because this is where the ability to attach and separate (Moursund & Erskine, 2004) is learned. Ideally, family life sits at the core of existence from birth to death (Madanes, 1982) because this can positively influence wellbeing. Bonding is a universal purpose of religion (Saroglou, 2021) and can be found at the familial level. Bowlby's (1969) seminal attachment theory is a useful lens for understanding the importance of secure bonding in the developmental years. This work provides an understanding of 'normal and pathological developmental processes' (Cortana & Marrone, 2008,

G. Harvey, *Fundamentalist Religious Childhoods and Adult Mental Health and Wellbeing*, https://doi.org/10.1007/978-3-032-20140-9_4

p. 19) based on the perspective that children are preprogrammed to form connections. Ainsworth and Wittig (1969) developed the theory further and identified secure, avoidant, and ambivalent insecure attachment styles. Main and Solomon (1990) then added an insecure, anxious, disorganised category later. The theory can be critiqued for the understanding of it as fixed rather than 'malleable' (Stein, 2017, p. 35), its unclear definition (Allen, 2016), the lack of recognition of genetic factors (Rutter, 2002), and for emphasising the mother–child relationship. This ignores bonds with other influential figures (Harris, 2002), including friends, adults, and leaders within fundamentalist religious organisations. There is a strong argument that the dynamics of the attachment figure relationship are stored by the child and become an internal working model (IWM) (Gillath et al., 2016; Golding & Hughes, 2012). Other writing supports the view that the mother who responds appropriately to the distress signals of their infant assists regulation (Rholes & Simpson, 2004) and supports the developing nervous system (Gerhardt, 2015) because:

> ... parents who are mindful of their children's needs and flexible in their interactions with them are literally assisting the neural wiring process in their children's brains (Thompson, 2010, p. 120).

Research on the parent–child bond within a fundamentalist religious family shows it to be a crucial consideration. One longitudinal study of early childhood revealed that the parent–child bond was shown to increase with religious mothers (Pearce & Axin, 1998, cited in Bartkowski et al., 2008) and fathers (Bartkowski et al., 2008). Similarly, an examination of longitudinal outcomes based on a national US survey (Bradford Wilcox, 1998) discovered a connection between the level of paternal religious involvement and engagement in one-to-one activities with their offspring. A large-scale survey of 3,124 conservative Protestant first-time fathers in the Fragile Families and Wellbeing study in America revealed that those who frequently attended religious community events reported greater involvement with their young children than those who did not (Petts, 2007).

Other studies have found that religion can 'detrimentally affect the bonding mechanism as explained in attachment theory' (Bowlby, 1969, cited in Simonic et al., 2013, p. 341) because religious parents tend to be less attuned to and communicative with their children (Simonic et al., 2013). Some literature states that the lack of a secure caregiver to whom the child can attach can lead to maladaptive relational coping behaviours, self-blame, and self-concept. It is unsurprising, then, that the children of religious addicts[1] can display similar co-dependent behaviours to those of the offspring of alcoholics (Arterburn & Felton, 1993), potentially contributing to an array of mental health issues (Walters, 1992, cited in Koenig & Larson, 2001). These findings support a child's need for close bonds by receiving constant, clear messages from the caregiver (Diamond & Marrone, 2006).

Some research has investigated the positive impact of religion on couples' relationships. One meta-analysis of over twelve studies carried out in the 1980s and 1990s (Mahoney et al., 2001) found a high correlation between regular attendance at a religious community and lower divorce rates, with more recent longitudinal research (Brown et al., 2008; Vaaler, 2009; Woods & Emery, 2002) having comparable findings. This is not surprising given that many highly religious people fervently believe in the nuclear family (Frisk et al., 2018, p. 69; McQueeny, 2009), and it suggests that religious parents' communal affiliation, where one can expect to be liked and well-treated (Grusec & Davidove, 2007, pp. 297–298), can facilitate a more stable family environment and healthy parent–child bonds.

Conversely, families at the fundamentalist end of the religious continuum, such as the Exclusive Brethren community, can become 'enmeshed', with the boundaries between the two becoming blurred so that the collectivist group then becomes family. Jenkinson (2019, p. 16) names this as 'confluence', like two tributaries merging into one river. This blends with Aguado's (2018) assertion that dysfunctional families lack healthy boundaries and function as a cult, implying that this is more likely within the dogmatic, legalistic, cognitive rigidity, (Yelderman,

[1] Religious addicts are those who engage in compulsive, mood-altering religious practices.

2018) and 'closed cognitive style' (Raschke, 1973, p. 339). *The parent–child bond can be detrimentally impacted by the adult's over-involvement in a group or primary bond with a deity figure.* In line with this, the likelihood of disorganised attachment bonds within groups (Stein & Russell, 2016) can result in the child living with the uncertainty of the caregiver being a safe sanctuary but also a threat because of parental over-involvement with leaders and the group (Stein, 2007). Consequently, the parent is not a secure base, and the child becomes angry, avoidant, or frozen, as the fight-flight-freeze mechanism is activated.

Bonding and Belonging in Fundamentalist Religious Communities

The perspective that the need for belonging is universally true for human beings, regardless of age, is elucidated by many writers (Lim et al., 2021; Sedgwick & Yonge, 2008). Some research has shown that being part of a faith community can have a positive impact on mental health (Blazer, 2009), with the frequency of attendance being a significant contributing factor (Jansen et al., 2010). For those of a religious persuasion, this can be met in synagogues, mosques, churches, and meeting halls. Diverse reasons for religious communal association exist and include shared relational support, help during times of personal challenge, and the continuation of family traditions. It is not surprising then that in the USA more people are affiliated to a religious organisation than to other groups (Putman, 2000) and that some non-religious, cultural Jews continue to observe customs and festivals and their links to the religious community (Hatch, 2015).

One of the benefits of the religious communal association for children can be the friendships forged with peers, despite often having no choice but to attend. 'The greatest thing in this church is the friends' (participant Sture cited in Frisk, 2018, p. 67). Some results have demonstrated that belonging to a religious community can encourage the development of a moral framework for young people (Ecklund & Lee, 2011; Laird et al., 2010, 2011), with one longitudinal study of over 600 African

American teenagers (Landor et al., 2011) showing that parental religious attendance to be inversely related to teenage risky sexual involvement.

It is important to acknowledge that communal religious involvement is only 'one element among many influences in childhood', with each child's upbringing being 'unique and idiosyncratic' (Birtwistle & Smith, 2012, p. 1). This challenges Frisk's (2018) declaration that accounts of growing up in the same religious group are often similar. Reality and memories also change over time (Yalom, 2017, p. 50), as can be seen when two accounts of an identical event differ (van Eck Duymaer van Twist, 2015).

Many writers argue that the need to belong applies to all human beings (Lim et al., 2021; Sedgwick & Yonge, 2008), regardless of age, gender, neurodiversity, race, ethnicity, culture, and sexuality etc. One way of satiating this is to belong to religious communities. Diverse reasons for this exist, and, as for adults, children can forge friendships with their peers, as demonstrated in some qualitative research reports. Holly grew up in the church that her father attended all his life. While not all co-researchers spoke about the dynamics of their religious group, they were all involved in the religious community to which their parents subscribed.

There was a sense of continuity for Eva, a second-generation adult (SGA), whose parents joined the Jehovah's Witnesses (JWs) before her birth. Eva's voice was warm as she shared her memories of the deep sense of belonging she had in childhood.

> *... so we did grow up together, all of us, and have quite good times. My Mum would do the children's parties, and there were some good times because we were part of a community. Very much a sense of belonging for a period of time, when we were infant children, we were all together, yes, those were probably quite good times ... I remember being part of something ... you know, very innocent and very wholesome.*

Holly found belonging with her peers at the church youth group and in her family.

> *I grew up in a very crazy, funny house with two sets of grandparents, a big house, and my grandparents lived there, and the church was, I would say, part of life. I think it was their only social activity.*

Similarly, Rupert, an only child who grew up within an Evangelical Baptist church, recalled his enjoyment of being involved in church life from a young age and spoke of the love, care, belonging, acceptance, friendship, and fun socialisation that he enjoyed. Sundays were special because he liked being at church and enjoyed the activities.

> *My church was a very warm and lively church. There was a lot of good care and teaching in it … In ways, there was a lot of love and care for one another; it was all very much family in one sense. We used to have socials, and you know it was a really great environment.*

Practical Support

This research also found that belonging to a religious community can be practically beneficial during difficult times. Holly's account of meals being provided when there was illness in her family supported this.

> *… if somebody was ill, you wouldn't have to cook for a whole week.*

This echoes the findings of self-reported cancer patients' experiences that revealed the importance of being given lifts to the hospital for treatment (Jim et al., 2015). Similarly, Rupert recounted the help he received from his church when his baby died. He also recalled the fear and anxiety of being the same age that his mother was when she had a mental breakdown. He told me that his Christian friends prayed for him, and the fear lifted and never returned. Invitations to those who live alone to share Shabbat or a Passover meal, taking a cake to welcome new neighbours, or supporting those sitting Shiva are an intrinsic part of Jewish religious communal life.

A Sense of Religious Lineage Adding to Bonding and Belonging

Religious lineage seemed to enhance belonging for some, especially Rupert, who was a multigenerational adult (MGA), with his church attendance and Christian faith continuing a long family tradition. He described this as 'a good Christian heritage' which has been passed on to subsequent generations. Hannah's story radiates a palpable sense of the positive health benefits that can result from religious communal belonging. This has been a priority throughout life, and she has passed this on to her children. Attending the synagogue and the celebration of religious festivals such as Passover, Rosh Hashanah, and Yom Kippur, with her family and friends, continues to be at the centre of life. Reciprocal support enables her to thrive as an adult. Holly also spoke proudly of her sense of religious lineage in relation to her father.

> *He was paraded in church on the day he was born, and the church was a vital element to my Dad.*

The importance of the continuance of transhistorical, transgenerational bonds with a religious community was evident in the stories of Hannah, Holly, and Rupert.

The Challenges of Enmeshment for Bonding and Belonging

The parent–child bond can be detrimentally impacted by an adult parent/parents' over-involvement with a group or deity figure. Some work acknowledges the likelihood of disorganised attachment within groups (Stein & Russell, 2016).

One of the reasons for this is the time-consuming nature of enmeshment. For example, 'the Laestadian (part of the Evangelical Lutheran Church of Finland), Mormon and JWs communities are often described as close-knit and highly demanding as they demand time, presence and participation on the part of their members' (Van Den Brandt &

Rantala, 2024, p. 229). An interview-based qualitative inquiry into the Abrahamic traditions interviewed the parents of twenty-four school-age children and discovered that, on average, religious activity was about twelve hours a week (Marks, 2004).

Holly reflected on her mixed feelings about her 'idiosyncratic' home environment, being proud of the practical ways in which her mother demonstrated her Christian faith.

> *I was proud of the drug addicts and sick people my Mum collected. Mum was a good and kind Christian … I think having a very sick Mum and an unattainable Dad and Mum that collected very ill people … because I then felt guilty that I should love everybody because I'm a good Christian. People used to think our house was the ideal house, but they didn't realise how difficult it was.*

Co-researcher Hannah felt that family and community life were separate but overlapped healthily. However, she acknowledged that the experiences of others within Judaism were not the same and that boundaries between family life and the religious group can become blurred when there is over-involvement.

One participant's story of growing up in the JWs and of her aunt, who, as a pioneer, knocked at people's doors and preached for over one hundred hours every month, illustrates the level of enmeshment that can exist. Eva also became a pioneer in her early twenties. She recalled how her father's service strained her parents' marriage because he was doing 'shepherding calls, preparing talks, and being involved in JW business' while her mother became lonely. She also spoke about the pressure.

> *… you know, we had to go on Tuesday night, we had to go on Thursday night. We had to go preaching … you weren't given a choice. It was oppressive, but without really knowing it, really realising it, unlike other children, I wanted to go, I fully embraced it, I wanted to be the good girl. I think I was looking for approval.*

Other participants accepted that their fundamentalist religious group demanded high levels of attendance at all events, which was very time-consuming. Francesca Alexandra recounted not having enough time to do her schoolwork because church attendance was required most evenings and weekends, and attendance was mandatory. Holly also talked about the pressure to attend church every Sunday and to prove that she was a true Christian by being very busy with church work. Anna emphasised that it was difficult to be oblivious to the pressure, by stating that it was not a hobby but involved church activities a couple of times a week with Girls' Brigade and Junior Christian Endeavour involvement, and several Sunday services.

Maya said that attendance at the mosque and madrassa was mandatory, although she did not have a sense of belonging anywhere. Hannah spoke warmly about her family's involvement, but she recognised the toll on family life that over-commitment exacted.

Anna described the intensity of the family and religious enmeshment in her childhood as the fact that:

> *.... we lived and breathed it.*

Francesca Alexandra's description of the relational dynamics in her family as inconsistent illustrates the confusion of some religious fundamentalist parenting.

> *Mum could be loving but also manipulative. Mum would devour me emotionally, enmesh me, eat me alive, emotional incest is what I'd call it ... Yet, when food was short, she'd give us the food and she'd be without ... a Mum that is trying to care.*

She also shared about her mother's reluctance to call a doctor when she was ill, so she stopped telling her parents when she was unwell because they would not have sought help. Her mother believed that God would heal a toothache, and consequently, dental treatment was withheld because of a distrust of dentists.

Francesca Alexandra experienced harsh discipline, telling me that she and her siblings were forced to smoke cigarettes when her parents suspected that they had stolen some. Her parents also disciplined them by:

> *... dressing up a cracker with pepper, dried peas and pretending it was mouldy bread, and we had to eat it.*

There was another side to her mother, however, who was a Sunday school teacher and deacon's wife because:

> *... she was being an obedient Christian wife.*

Francesca Alexandra bonded with her father, and he was her safe parent for sixty to seventy per cent of the time.

> *Safe in terms of being funny, being nice to be around, but there was this percentage that actually he wasn't, but just using the safe percentage for that part, he gave me enough to buffer me a bit, really.*

The parenting that Francesca Alexandra received was inconsistent.

There were many challenges in the mother-daughter relationship for Eva.

> *She wasn't able to let me get close or to accept me, so that was sad because it ruined any chance of us being close, really. After all, she was such a fighter that she fought everybody. Right at the end, when she became ill and she was relying on me, that's when she realised I was there for her, so we did have those two years or so. I spent a lot of time by her side in the nursing home, so that was her making peace in a way, because we hadn't really done much together, not when I was growing up, you know.*

It is clear that while some of the co-researchers were able to bond and have a sense of belonging in the religious community and family, which could potentially benefit wellbeing in adulthood, this was not everyone's experience.

The Loss of Bonding and Belonging in a Religious Family and Community

Mytton's (2013) research revealed that members leave high-demand groups in three different ways. Some are disfellowshipped (16 per cent), while others leave because of others' decisions (18 per cent), with 67 per cent choosing to leave. The latter category is members with 'unresolved doubts and dissonance' (Coates, 2013, p. 314) who can no longer resolve them by denial and avoidance. This is backed up by the findings of a research study of twenty-three former members of eleven cults, with the participants leaving 'as a solution to the stress and emotional exhaustion of membership' (Coates, 2013, p. 314). This was true for co-researcher Eva, who, despite being a baptised member, became depressed and felt hopeless when she thought she was in the JWs for the rest of her life. Following allegations of sexual abuse within the organisation, and meeting with the elders to confess that she was in a relationship with someone she'd met at work, she left.

> *I walked out of there and thought I don't want this anymore.*

She told me that people who chose to leave were judged to be:

> *... very bad and very worldly, oh, they've gone out of the truth, they're not in the truth anymore, they've become worldly, they've got worldly friends, worldly tendencies ... they have the spirit of the world.*

In Eva's words:

> *I lost everything; everyone shunned*[2] *me. Having been in the organisation all of my life ... They told everyone not to communicate with me. I think when I left, I had this notion that I could close the door on it and start a new life, and I mean, I suppose there's no other way to approach it because you've made a decision. But two years of no contact with anybody, two quite difficult years, really.*

---

[2] Shunning is a literal form of 'dispensing of existence' (Lifton, 1989) adopted by the Jehovah's Witnesses and other religious groups to punish apostates.

This haunting statement by Eva is confirmed in Mytton's (2013) findings, which revealed that 53 per cent of those who left lost contact with close family, increasing to 76 per cent when extended family was included. Noticeably, 66 per cent of the 250+ participants were no longer in contact with their parents, while over 90 per cent had experienced substantial loss since exiting the high-demand fundamentalist religious group.

Some texts acknowledge the negative prejudice displayed towards ex-members through shunning and ostracism. This 'universal way of punishing non-compliance' (Harvey, 2020, p. 7) discards people (Lifton, 1989), with non-believers being ousted from a group, excluded, and ignored, with existing social ties severed (Gutgsell, 2017, p. 18). Ostracism is one of the 'unethical, manipulative or coercive techniques of persuasion and control' (Lagone, 1993, p. 4) required for the system to remain sealed in terms of 'the marble edifice' (Jenkinson, 2016, p. 226) and the group free from 'contradictory beliefs and immoral behaviours' (Zieman, 2018, p. 5). This in turn, enables 'milieu control, mystical manipulation, demand for purity, confession, sacred science, loaded language, doctrine over person and dispensing of existence' (Lifton, 1989, cited in Jenkinson, 2023, p.190) to continue within the group, with the leader's god-like authority permitting a shunning edict to be issued that 'everyone in the group is required to follow … friends – family – even, to a degree, members of one's own household' (Zieman, 2018, p. xiv). Practically, ostracism is about what behaviours people refuse to do with the person viewed as unclean, for example, no eye contact, not responding, and not sitting at the same table.

Mandatory shunning manipulates by utilising polarised opposite techniques to 'love-bombing' (Singer, 2003, p. 114), which commonly seduces someone into a group in the first place because 'they are made to feel special, loved, among newfound friends and a part of something unique' (Lalich & Tobias, 2006, p. 25). *Shunning, however, 'affects four fundamental human needs; the need for belonging, self-esteem, control and meaningful existence'* (Gutgsell, 2017, p. 6). No wonder that Zieman (2018, p. xii) argues that it 'is one of the worst things that can happen to a human'. It has also been called 'ubiquitous' (Zieman, 2018, p. 4), 'a social death, an insidious form of psychological torture' (Zieman, 2018,

p. 4), 'a vile practice' (Zieman, 2018, p. 3) and the New Testament equivalent of stoning someone to death. Moreover, this is a permanent punishment unless the person is willing to reintegrate and fully adopt the thoughts, beliefs, and practices of the group again. Even then, the re-joining process can take many months and sometimes longer' (Freestone, 2018, p. 4), and it is therefore not surprising that 'the prospect of being shunned is another immense barrier for those considering leaving' (Stein, 2017, p. 175).

Members can be forced to exit a religious group if they start to question, behave in inappropriate ways, or refuse to conform. The JWs are the religious group that is most recognised for disfellowshipping baptised members who do not comply with the strict moral code, with three of the church elders judging the seriousness of the breach. Some members exit the group via a written resignation known as dissociating, but this can also be imposed upon members who voice disagreement or fail to be obedient. The JW community shuns those exiting, which has been described as 'the social death' (Ransom et al., 2021, p. 2458).

In this fourth chapter, it has become apparent that the innate human need for connection through bonding and belonging can be met in fundamentalist religious families and communities. Conversely, noncompliance and questioning can result in being ejected from the group and rejected by family and friends. This is known as a living bereavement, which is one of the loneliest grief experiences a human being can experience and can greatly challenge both physical and mental health.

References

Aguado, J. F. (2018). How a dysfunctional family functions like a cult. *ICSA Today.*, *9*(3), 2–7.

Ainsworth, M. I. S., & Wittig, B. A. (1969). *Attachment and the exploratory behaviour of one-year-olds in a strange situation*. Methuen.

Allen, B. (2016). A radical idea: A call to eliminate attachment disorder and attachment theory from the clinical lexicon. *Evidence-Based Practice in Child and Adolescent Mental Health, 1*(1), 60–71. https://doi.org/10.1080/23794925.2016.1172945

Arterburn, S., & Felton J. (1993). *Faith that hurts, faith that heals.* Thomas Nelson.

Bartkowski, J. P., Xu, X., & Levin, M. L. (2008). Religion and child development: Evidence from the Early Childhood Longitudinal Study. *Social Science Research, 37*, 18–36. https://doi.org/10.1016/j.ssresearch.2007.02.001

Birtwistle, L., & Smith, L. (2012). *Children growing-up with religion: Ten narratives explored.* York Publishing Services.

Blazer, D. G. (2009). Religion, spirituality, and mental health: What we know and why this is a tough topic to research. *The Canadian Journal of Psychiatry, 54*(5), 281–291.

Bowlby, J. (1969). *Attachment and loss Volume 1: Attachment.* Basic Books.

Bradford Wilcox, W. (1998). Conservative Protestant childrearing: Authoritarian or authoritative? *American Sociological Review, 63*, 796–809. https://doi.org/10.2307/2657502

Brown, E., Orbuch, T. L., & Bauermeister, J. A. (2008). Religiosity and marital stability among Black American and White American couples. *Family Relations, 57*, 186–197. https://doi.org/10.1111/j.1741-3729.2008.00493.x

Coates, D. D. (2013). Disaffiliation from a new religious movement: The importance of self and others in exit. *Symbolic Interaction, 36*(3), 313–334. https://doi.org/10.1002/SYMB.60

Collins English Dictionary. (2019). https://www.collinsdictionary.com/dictionary/english/abrahamic.

Cortana, D., & Marrone, M. (2008). *Attachment theory and the psychoanalytic process.* Whurr.

Diamond, N., & Marrone, M. (2006). *Attachment and intersubjectivity.* Whurr.

Ecklund, E. H., & Lee, K. S. (2011). Atheists and agnostics negotiate religion and family. *Journal for the Scientific Study of Religion, 50*(4), 728–743.

Freestone, N. (2018). *Becoming 'part of the world'. Helping former Jehovah's Witnesses adjust to life outside the religion.* https://www.jwfacts.com/pdf/freestone-jw-therapy-2018.pdf.

Frisk, L. (2018). Growing up in controversial minority religions: Constructions of childhood. In L. Frisk, S. Nilsson, & P. Akerback (Eds.), *Children in minority religions. Growing up in controversial religious groups* (pp. 64–94). Equinox.

Gerhardt, S. (2015). *Why love matters: How affection shapes a baby's brain.* Routledge.

Gillath, O., Karantzas, G. C., & Fraley, R. C. (2016). *Adult attachment: A concise introduction to theory and research.* Elsevier.

Golding, K. S., & Hughes, D. A. (2012). *Creating loving attachments.* Jessica Kingsley.
Grusec, J. E., & Davidov, M. (2007). Socialization in the family: The roles of parents. In J. E. Grusec & P. D. Hastings (Eds.), *Handbook of socialization: Theory and research* (pp. 284–308). Guildford Press.
Gutgsell, J. (2017). *A loving provision? How former Jehovah's Witnesses experience shunning.* Master's thesis, Vrije Universiteit Brussels, Brussels. https://saysorry.org/wp-content/uploads/2019/09/shunning-and-disfellowshipping-in-jehovahswitnesses-by-j-gutgsell.pdf
Harris, R. (2002). *Christ-centred therapy: Empowering the self.* Routledge.
Harvey, G. (2020). Ostracism. *ICSA Today, 11*(3), 7–9.
Hatch, T. G. (2015). *Mishpacha in the America Diaspora: An exploratory study of highly-involved Jewish families.* PhD thesis, Louisiana State University. http://digitalcommons.lsu.edu/gradschool_dissertations/519
Jansen, K., Motley, R., & Hovey, J. (2010). Anxiety, depression, and students' religiosity. *Mental Health, Religion & Culture, 13*(3), 267–271.
Jenkinson, G. (2016). *Freeing the authentic self: Phases of recovery and growth from an abusive cult experience.* PhD thesis, University of Nottingham. https//.www.eprints/Nottingham/ac.uk/25707/1/161202/GillianJenkinson/FinalThesis.USE.pdf
Jenkinson, G. (2019). *Post-cult counselling workbook. A guide for your recovery and growth.* Hope Valley Counselling.
Jenkinson, G. (2023). *Walking free from the trauma of coercive*. Routledge.
Jim, H. S. L., Pustejovsky, J. E., Park, C. L., Danhauer, S. C., Sherman, A. C., Fitchett, G., Merluzzi, T. V., Munoz, A. R., George, L., Snyder, M. A., & Salsman, J. M. (2015). *Religion, spirituality, and physical health in cancer patients: A meta-analysis.* wileyonlinelibrary.com. https://doi.org/10.1002/cncr.29353
Koenig, H. G., & Larson, D. B. (2001). Religion and mental health: Evidence for an association. *International Review of Psychiatry, 13*, 67–78. https://doi.org/10.1080/09540260124661
Lagone, M. (Ed.). (1993). *Recovery from cults: Help for victims of psychological and spiritual abuse.* Norton.
Laird, R., Marks, L. D., & Marrero, M. (2011). Religiosity, self-control and antisocial behavior: Religiosity as a promotive and protective factor. *Journal of Applied Developmental Psychology, 32*, 78–85. https://doi.org/10.1016/j.appdev.2010.12.003
Laird, R. D., Marrero, M. D., & Marks, L. D. (2010). Adolescent religiosity as a protective factor for delinquency: Review of evidence and a conceptual

framework for future research. In O. Sahin, & J. Maier, (Eds). *Delinquency: Causes, reduction, and prevention.* Nova Science.

Lalich, J., & Tobias, M. (2006). *Take back your life: Recovering from cults and abusive relationships.* Bay Tree.

Landor, A., Simons, L. G., Simons, R. L., Brody, G. H., & Gibbons, F. X. (2011). The role of religiosity in the relationship between parents, peers, and adolescent risky sexual behavior. *Journal of Youth and Adolescence, 40*(3), 296–309. https://doi.org/10.1007/s10964-010-9598-2

Lifton, R. J. (1989). *Thought reform and the psychology of totalism. A study of "brainwashing" in China.* The University of North Carolina Press.

Lim, M. H., Allen, K. A., Furlong, M. J., Craig, H., & Smith, D. C. (2021). Introducing a dual continuum model of belonging and loneliness. *Australian Journal of Psychology, 72*(1), 81–86. https://doi.org/10.1080/00049530.2021.1883411

Madanes, C. (1982). *Strategic family therapy.* Amorrortu editores.

Mahoney, A., Pargament, K. I., Tarakeshwar, N., & Swank, A. B. (2001). Religion in the home in the 1980s and 1990s: A meta-analytic review and conceptual analyses of links between religion, marriage, and parenting. *Journal of Family Psychology, 15*, 559–596.

Main, M., & Solomon, J. (1990). Procedures for identifying infants as disorganized/disorientated during the Ainsworth Strange situation. In M. T. Greenberg, D. Cicchetti, & E. M. Cummings (Eds.), *Attachment in the preschool years: Theory, research and interventions* (pp. 121–160). The University of Chicago Press.

Marks, L. (2004). Sacred practices in high religious families: Christian, Jewish, Mormon, and Muslim perspectives. *Family Process, 43*(2), 217–231. https://doi.org/10.1111/j.1545-5300.2004.04302007.x

McQueeny, K. (2009). "We are all God's children, y'all": Race, gender, and sexuality in lesbian and gay-affirming congregations. *Social Problems, 56*, 151–173.

Moursund, J. P., & Erskine, R. G. (2004). *Integrative psychotherapy: The art and science of relationship.* Brookes Cole.

Mytton, J. (2013). *Second-generation adult survivors of the Hales Exclusive Brethren: Mental health, childhood sexual abuse and interpersonal problems.* Paper presented at The International Cultic Studies Association Annual Conference, Trieste, Italy.

Petts, R. J. (2007). Religious participation, religious affiliation, and engagement with children among fathers experiencing the birth of a new child. *Journal of Family Issues, 28*, 1139–1161. https://doi.org/10.1177/0192513X07300788

Putman, R. (2000). *Bowling alone: The collapse and revival of American community.* Simon and Schuster.
Ransom, H. J., Monk, R. L., & Heim, D. (2021). Grieving the living: The social death of former Jehovah's Witnesses. *Journal of Religion and Health, 61*, 2458–2480. https://doi.org/10.1007/s10943-020-01156-8
Raschke, G. (1973). Dogmatism and committed and consensual religiosity. *Journal for the Scientific Study of Religion, 12*(3), 339–344.
Rholes, W. S., & Simpson, J. A. (2004). *Attachment theory and religiosity: A summary of empirical research with implications for counselling Christian clients.* Guilford.
Rutter, M. (2002). Nature, nurture, and development: From evangelism through science towards policy and practice. *Child Development, 72*(1), 1–21. https://doi.org/10.1111/1467-8624.00388
Saroglou, V. (2021). *The psychology of religion.* Routledge.
Sedgwick, M. G., & Yonge, O. (2008). We're in it, we're a team, we're family means a sense of belonging. *Rural and Remote Health, 8*, 1021. http://www.rrh.org.au/.
Simonic, B., Mandelj, T. R., & Novsak, R. (2013). Religious-related abuse in the family. *Journal of Family Violence, 28*, 339–349. https://doi.org/10.1007/s10896-013-9508-y
Singer, M. T. (2003). *Cults in our midst: The continuing fight against their hidden menace.* Jossey-Bass.
Stein, A. (2007). *Attachment, networks and discourse in extremist political organisations. A comparative case study.* PhD thesis, University of Minnesota. https://www.academia/edu/1971678/Attachment_networks_and_discourse_in_extremist_political_organizations_A_comparative_case_study
Stein, A. (2017). *Terror, love & brainwashing. Attachment in cults and totalitarian systems.* Routledge.
Stein, A., & Russell, M. (2016). Attachment theory and post-cult recovery. *Therapy Today, 27*(7), 18–21.
Thompson, C. (2010). *Anatomy of the soul. Surprising connections between neuroscience and spiritual practices that can transform your life and relationship.* Tyndale House.
Vaaler, M. L., Ellison, C. G., & Powers, D. A. (2009). Religious influences on the risk of marital dissolution. *Journal of Marriage and Family, 71*(4), 917–934. https://doi.org/10.1111/j.1741-3737.2009.00644.x
Van den Brandt, N., & Rantala, T. (2024). Gendered and embodied un/learning among women disengaging from faith in the UK and Finland. *Approaching Religion, 14*(2), 224–239.

Van Eck Duymaer van Twist. (2015). *Perfect children: Growing up on the religious fringe.* Oxford University Press. https://doi.org/10.1093/acprof.oso/9780199827787.001.0001

Woods, L. N., & Emery, R. E. (2002). The cohabitation effects on divorce: Causation or selection? *Journal of Divorce and Remarriage, 37*, 101–119. https://doi.org/10.1300/J087v37n03_06

Yalom, I. D. (2017). *Becoming myself. A psychiatrist's memoir.* Little, Brown.

Yelderman, L. A. (2018). Cognitive rigidity explains the relationship between religious fundamentalism and insanity defence attitudes. *Mental Health, Religion & Culture, 21*(7), 686–697. https://doi.org/10.1080/13674676.2018.1551340

Zieman, B. (2018). *Shunned: A survival guide.* Amazon.

5

The Gaining of Knowledge About Religious Matters from a Young Age, and Foundational Beliefs and Practices Enabling Resilience

The Gaining of Knowledge About Religious Matters from a Young Age

All of the co-researchers were 'trained' (US Legal Inc, 2019) in the single religious tradition to which their caregivers subscribed. Such training originates from the common beliefs or 'creeds' (Greenberg & Witztum, 2001, p. 37) that form a foundational connection with other believers in that religious community. Research outcomes consistently demonstrate that the way that religious parents raise their children is usually based on their belief system (Chen & VanderWeele, 2018, p. 2355), and views about a deity figure are based on the teachings from the holy texts relevant to that religion. It is claimed that if such beliefs are continued into adulthood, they could aid 'emotional stability and resolution of mental conflict' (Hand, 2002, cited in Koenig & Larson, 2001, p. 67).

God (Allah) is the most important core concept within Western religion, and this concurs with the monomorphic view of God within Abrahamic religious expressions (De Sondy et al., 2021, p. 1). One paper that had 585 participants from Protestant, Catholic, and Jewish backgrounds, as well as some from so-called minority religions, reveals

G. Harvey, *Fundamentalist Religious Childhoods and Adult Mental Health and Wellbeing*, https://doi.org/10.1007/978-3-032-20140-9_5

perspectives of God as 'companiable, benevolent, wrathful, with omniness and potentially present' (Gorsuch, 1968, pp. 56–64). By comparison, another qualitative study of 30 African American couples finds that beliefs about God's nature as loving and a source of strength in difficult times, with marriage and family viewed as designed by God (Marks et al., 2012). Other studies (Burr et al., 2012; Dollahite et al., 2012; Goodman & Dollahite, 2006; Goodman et al., 2013) also show positive beliefs about God. Children are known to take on the beliefs, emotions, and boundaries of the family and larger systems in which they are embedded. An abundance of general theories exist about child development, including social learning theory (Bandura, 1977) and psychosocial development theory (Erikson, 1950), and it is generally agreed that Piaget's (1936) work on cognitive developmental theory is foundational to such thinking. Piaget's work proposes that a child's cognitive comprehension of a deity figure increases in stages, with more concrete and intricate images evolving as the child grows older. This is helpful for understanding that children take on their parental and group beliefs, although it fails to consider that each child's religious development will be different (Hood et al., 2018) and 'unique and idiosyncratic' (Birtwistle & Smith, 2012, p. 1). There is also evidence to support the developmental stages of God comprehension thinking in Ladd et al.'s (1998) pictorial research of 968 US children, age range 3–18 years, which indicates a linear increase in the use of symbolism and God images developing in stages as proposed by Piagetian theory. This suggests that if a child's conceptualisation of God is positive, proximity behaviours towards the deity as a substitute object are possible (Bowlby, 1969; Main, 1990). This is backed by Granqvist's (2014) idea that God can become a symbolic, surrogate attachment figure who supplies security, protection, guidance, and reliability (Kaufman, 1981, p. 67). Other research suggests that Allah can become an attachment figure for children growing up with adult Islamic beliefs (Bagher et al., 2013; Miner et al., 2014). Some Christian writers (Houser & Welch, 2013) take this further by suggesting that positive belief in and attachment to God is an a priori feature of healthy human bonding, which is made more possible by caregivers displaying godly characteristics (Ashley, 2015; Steege, 2010).

Within religious fundamentalism, an image of an authoritative, punishing God will often be painted (Heimlich, 2011). The opportunity for a deity figure to be a secure base is questionable if the deity is viewed as punishing and wrathful. Similarly, the 'omni-ness' of God (Gorsuch, 1968, pp. 56–64) as all-seeing and all-knowing might be a terrifying substitute attachment person. This is symbolically clarified in the following quotation about patient Karl's mother.

> I lived in a glass house in which my mother could look at any time. In a glass house, however, you cannot conceal anything without giving yourself away, except by hiding it under the ground. And then you cannot see it yourself either. (cited in Miller, 1987, p. 21)

While some children might turn to God as a safe attachment during difficulties (Beck & McDonald, 2004), this is unlikely when a child is terrified of God.

Beliefs About Children in Fundamentalist Religious Families and Communities

Integral to the intergenerational and intercultural transmission of religious matters are beliefs about children. This influences the way that children are treated, as demonstrated in the research with new orthodox Jewish mothers, which discovered the belief that 'children are a trust from God, and parenthood a sacred responsibility' (Hatch, 2015, p. 36), so that offspring are cherished. Some commentators argue that within fundamentalist religious groups, children are often seen as important, so parents are committed to their children, spending much time with them: 'the raising of offspring seems, at times, to be a life project' (Frisk, 2018a, p. 70). Conversely, Winell (2020a) maintains that Christianity has a low view of children, the foundational reason being the way they are negatively objectified in the Bible and sacrificed in some Old Testament stories.

In some fundamentalist religious groups, such as the JWs, youngsters are viewed as inferior with a hierarchy of God, father, mother, and then children (Frisk, 2018a). Differing beliefs about children were exemplified in one ethnographic project (Strhan, 2017), which researched how children were treated in two different British evangelical Christian churches. In the charismatic evangelical church, children were welcomed and included in activities, and in comparison, the conservative evangelical church kept children separate and less visible, with expectations of obedience to their parents and male leaders. Yet, in both churches, children learned about religious matters from a young age. Rupert not only gained knowledge of Christianity from childhood but also developed his faith from an early age. He became a Christian at seven years and was baptised by immersion in his early teens because he recognised that he was a sinner who needed God's love. Holly was taught about Christian matters at home, at her church and youth group. The nature of what she learned is evident in her description of her parents as:

> *... strongly evangelical Bible-believing Christians who were teetotal.*

Similarly, Eva's early learning about faith matters took place at home and the Kingdom Hall, where she normalised her learning about religion.

Hannah gained knowledge about religious matters in the synagogue and at home. She went to a Jewish primary school where teaching about religious matters was included. Her upbringing was different from that of the other participants in that she was able to question and be independent and self-governing. She recognised that at the fundamentalist end of Judaism, much more dogmatic and literal forms of religion mean that children are trained in the ultra-orthodox way of life, where conforming is mandatory. Anna believes that she started to learn about religious matters pre-birth because her mother prayed for her when she was still in the womb. What she experienced at home was replicated in her friends' families because they were all members of the same church. She described what she was taught.

> *Dogmatic, very clear-cut and literal, with no space to move. We lived and breathed it.*

What she learned was a direct replica of the teaching that her parents received and their beliefs about God. This connects with Chen and VanderWeele's (2018) assertion that children are commonly brought up with their parents' influential religious perspectives.

The Intergenerational and Intercultural Transmission of Religious Matters

The intergenerational transmission of religious beliefs and teachings throughout the Abrahamic traditions is viewed as vital according to Lees and Horwarth (2009). Scourfield et al.'s (2017) perspective that the intergenerational transmission of beliefs is a higher priority for Islamic parents than for Christian ones appears to be a sweeping generalisation. Jewish parents believe that passing on religious beliefs is an honour that should not be delegated to outsiders (Green, 1905, with parents given most of the responsibility, thus honouring the Jewish value of v'shinantam l'vanecha[1] (Marks et al., 2017). The importance of the parent–child bond in the intergenerational transmission of beliefs is highlighted in Okagaki and Bevis's (1999) work, which used a scale measure to quantify the warmth of the mother–child relationship, judged to be importantly influential on the degree to which parental beliefs were accepted by a young person. Other texts also credibly note that the intergenerational transmission of beliefs is not 'a cold-blooded technical process of cognitive downloading' (Berliner & Sarró, 2007, p. 10) but that it happens naturally within cultural settings.

This idealistic picture of religious parenting is challenged by the recognition that, although one literature review found that studies of religious manipulation in the family setting are rare (Simonic et al., 2013), emotional abuse and neglect exist, facilitated by parental religious beliefs (Bottoms et al., 1995). Some concerns have been raised about the corrective strategies used in religious households, mainly conservative Protestant families (Bartkowski et al., 2008), with physical and sexual child abuse being vindicated by scripture (Horton & Williamson, 1998).

[1] The Jewish value of v'shinantam l'vanecha is 'you shall teach your children'.

Frisk (2018b) asserts that some consider that the Bible supports the physical disciplining of children to correct them. She provides an example in the Twelve Tribes[2] and the use of a little stick to spank young children as a disciplinary practice. Her life-story qualitative findings reveal this as a common practice among ex-member participants of the JWs and The Family International/Children of God[3]:

> If you told the child to do something three times and they still did not obey you, then they were to be punished. If they tried to escape, they should be whipped on the legs three or four times. If they were disobedient and rude, they should be slapped around the head ten times. The belt should be used ten times. First, you should explain to the children, but never angrily, 'You have been disobedient, so now you will get ten lashes on the buttocks with the belt.' And they were not allowed to scream. Afterwards, they should be given a hug, and then the parents were to pray with them. (participant Bea, ex-member of TFI, Frisk, 2018b, p. 211)

This connects with Heimlich's (2011) accusation that fundamentalist authoritarian parenting within Christianity is based on a foundational obsession with child submission based on the doctrine of original sin[4] where everything outside of narrow Christianity is prohibited as being of the world. This includes academic study, politics, fashion, and the arts. Winell (2020a) maintains that Christianity has a low view of children. The belief is that children are sinners and that their will needs to be broken so that their selfish nature is controlled (Frisk, 2018b).

> Many parents and grandparents see it as their duty to impart the teachings of their faith to their children. In some belief systems that involve having as many children as possible to raise in the traditions of the faith. (Marich, 2024, p. 29)

---

[2] The Twelve Tribes is a controversial religious movement within Christianity.

[3] Another minority religion within Christianity.

[4] This doctrine states that all humans are born sinful due to 'the fall' of Adam and Eve, and that Jesus Christ suffered for the sins of humankind to atone for their sins. This belief affects how many Christians appraise the world, themselves, and their children (Heimlich, 2011, p. 99).

This image of love is not always replicated in the literature or in some of the co-researchers' stories. Francesca Alexandra described the unhealthy way that she was taught.

> *My mother grabbed hold of the rigidity of fundamentalism, which meant that she would have fed it to me in my growing-up years through the lens of her illness, highly neurotic and, I suspect, psychotic at times, being very judgmental and perceiving anyone who did not agree with her as a threat.*

Anna spoke about the forced nature of the parental transmission of religion in her home, which resonated with Maya's story of being steeped in the religion of Islam in her growing-up years, as she was taught by her grandparents, with whom she mainly lived, by her mother, and by being forced to attend the mosque.

While the benefit of learning about religious matters from a young age emerged as a strong similarity for participants in the findings, it is again clear that this was not true for all, as some were traumatised by the beliefs and behaviour. The forced nature of the intergenerational and intercultural transmission of religious matters, including physical, emotional, and psychological punishment for some, was traumatic, while others felt safe and loved in their family and the wider religious group.

Foundational Beliefs and Practices Enabling Resilience

> To believe is to be human; it undergirds our ability to imagine, experiment, relate to others and the world. (McGrath, 2025, p. 9)

Belief in the Holy Books

Young people growing up within a fundamentalist religious environment are taught from the holy texts relevant to that religious system. These teachings are not restricted to portraying a deity (God), because the Abrahamic traditions are known as 'scriptural religions', as their holy texts offer doctrine, meaning, and guidance (Yip et al., 2011). Although all these traditions acknowledge the Hebrew Bible as foundational, the Tanakh for Jews, the Qur'an for Muslims, and the Christian Bible are now very different guides (De Sondy et al., 2021). Belief in the appropriate holy book is so great that children will be familiarised with it from a young age, often learning portions of it by rote. Heimlich (2011) argues that the King James version of the Bible is 'a product of authoritarianism', with literal interpretation of those parts concerned with the sacrifice of children, for example, being terrifyingly traumatising for a young person (Heimlich, 2011). Some teachings from the holy books, such as about God's punishment, devils, or jinns,[5] or a literal belief in purgatory, hell, and eternal damnation, can lead to 'apeirophobia: the fear of eternity' (Azarian, 2016). Winell (2020b) also highlights the fact that some of the harmful doctrines within Christianity to which a child might be exposed from a young age, teaching about salvation, and that the self is bad and needs to be saved, for example, can negatively impact identity and lead to low self-worth and difficulties with decision-making later in life. She also points out that teaching about the 'end times',[6] 'the rapture',[7] and eternal consequences can trigger anxiety, phobias, and nightmares for a long time. While both Winell (2020b) and Heimlich (2011) raise significant points regarding the potential danger of such indoctrination,[8] together with critical thinking not being allowed, these are perspectives that solely concentrate on Christianity and suggest some bias because they do not consider other Abrahamic traditions.

In addressing the important matter of the influence of the holy texts on parenting practices, Holden and Williamson (2014) state that while none of the scriptures are child-rearing manuals, within Islam, both the

[5] Satan and devils are known within Islam as jinns.

[6] The 'end times' is the term used to denote the belief that the world will end in a cataclysmic event.

[7] The word 'rapture' means 'removal' in Christian scripture, principally associated with 1 Thessalonians 4:17. Some believe that Christians will be removed from the earth before the worst of the predicted events of the end of the world occur, and they call this the rapture.

[8] Indoctrination is when children are socialised into a religious belief system from a young age where compliance with the taught doctrines is necessary to survival.

Qur'an and the[9] Hadith have passages about the treatment of children and what is required of parents to pass on their religious beliefs and practices. Holden and Williamson (2014) also say that within the Christian scriptures, there is little direct guidance on raising children apart from in three of Paul's epistles (Ephesians, Colossians, and Timothy)[10] where children are exhorted to obey their parents, and fathers are urged not to exasperate them but to bring them up within the faith.

As has been evident, Francesca Alexandra's foundational beliefs, values, and practices acquired in childhood were often conveyed in a strict and punishing way, including the need to learn some Bible passages by rote. It is not surprising that her view of God was terrifying, and that he was constantly trying to catch her out, backed up by verses that stated that sin would be found out.

What is barely recognised in the literature is that socialisation is powerfully influential on a young person's belief system, and within fundamentalism, an image of an authoritative, punishing God is often painted (Heimlich, 2011). Similarly, the 'omni-ness' of God (Gorsuch, 1968, pp. 56–64), as all-seeing and all-knowing, might be a terrifying substitute attachment person. This is metaphorically stated in the glasshouse quotation.

Co-researcher Francesca Alexandra describes her experience:

> *... scripture was rammed down the throat, and it was about frightening people, hellfire ... and I was shamed for being me, for having needs and desires. For existing. So probably like, you know, we end up denying our thoughts, feelings and denying pleasure because it could involve the world.*

She was taught that the world was dangerous and full of traps that could send her to hell, as God was always waiting to catch her out.

> *God was terrifying, trying to catch me out ... He's all-knowing ... so be sure your sins will find you out, we were taught that in Sunday School, again*

[9] The Hadith are a collection of sayings, actions, and silent approvals of the Prophet Muhammed, the second most important source of Islamic law and moral guidance after the Qur'an.

[10] New Testament chapters of the Christian Bible.

another reason to be hypervigilant because … you'll be looking over your shoulder.

In addition, she became fearful and was terrified by the teaching, particularly the indoctrination around the second coming of Christ.[11]

Well, you might be wicked, so you might come home from school, and your parents aren't there, so they've been raptured. Good girls will be raptured, we'll go up to heaven when Jesus comes, and if you haven't been good, then you'll be left behind …

Despite the inappropriate ways in which Francesca Alexandra was taught Christian concepts, her story confirms the assertion that if a child's understanding of God is positive, proximity behaviour towards the deity as a substitute object is possible (Bowlby, 1969, p. 313; Main, 1990), enabling God to become a symbolic, surrogate attachment figure (Granqvist, 2014) supplying security, protection, guidance, and reliability (Kaufman, 1981, p. 67). Her bonding with the Almighty was linked to the unavailability of her mother.

While some children might turn to their God as a safe attachment during difficulties (Beck & McDonald, 2004, p. 1010), this is unlikely when a child believes in an all-seeing, ever-present deity from whom there is no escape. Participant Anna spoke about such teaching, terrifying her. Marich (2024, p. 41) describes the long-term effects on her.

The vengeful bogeyman of an Evangelical God that my father raised me to fear is still creeping around somewhere.

[11] The second coming of Christ means for some Christians the moment of Christ's reappearance on earth; for others it is a general term covering everything associated with the final judgement and the creation of a new heaven and earth.

Religious Practices

It is widely recognised that religious practices can serve as coping mechanisms, with Rupert explicitly acknowledging the positive influence of prayer. Some literature reveals that if religious practices are continued into adulthood, they can facilitate resilience and 'emotional stability and resolution of mental conflict' (Hand, 2002, cited in Koenig & Larson, 2001). Co-researcher Holly mentioned a Christian client she was working with who was having a difficult time, but it was 'worship and stuff ... the joy of the Lord is my strength' that gave her resilience.

Hannah described the healthy consistency of her religious upbringing.

> *I was brought up in a very independent way ... and had a Jewish education for my primary years, although not for secondary school ... I was very immersed in Judaism from a very early age ... e.g. Shabbat meals, so every weekend the meals were absolutely sacred and still are now. I grew up in a pretty practising Jewish home welcoming the Shabbat through the lighting of candles, usually by the woman in the household, but I was never made to feel that I'd be punished for keeping Shabbat or not, I think my parents would have been highly disappointed and I would have felt enormously guilty, but at the end of the day it was my own decision and the same is true for the next generation, my children, I'd rather they felt they'd come to their own decisions for the right reasons than to keep something for the sake of keeping it because then that would veer into the idea of abuse.*

Throughout life, she has integrated religious practices like Shabbat, which is like the Christian sabbath on a Sunday except that it lasts for twenty-five hours, starting on Friday an hour before sunset, and ending on Saturday evening at sunset (the timing varies between summer and winter). Shabbat observers do not use transport during the observance time, so it is much easier to live within walking distance of the synagogue and friends. Hannah regularly attended the synagogue where a different portion of the Sefer Torah (the parchment scrolls of the Old Testament) was read. She views Shabbat as a day of rest that supports mental health and wellbeing, and would like to see a day of rest implemented nationally. Describing the lighting of five candles for each of her family members to welcome Shabbat, she stated:

I feel quite emotional ... that settled feeling of rest.

Religious Rituals

Religious ritual can aid resilience because it is:

> structured behaviour, usually public, that acts out the patterns of engagement with the religion's supernatural agents. (De Sondy et al., 2021, p. 6)

Engaging in frequent prayer and Bible-reading helps manage voices for some people with schizophrenia, and higher levels of religiosity have correlated with increased compliance in taking prescribed medication (Mohr et al., 2006).

The statement that ritual is detested by fundamentalist Christians (Ineichen, 2019) is contradicted by the example Stott (2017) provides of enduring the very long prayer meetings in her Exclusive Brethren (EB) childhood, where she was expected to be compliantly quiet for hours. In practice, children growing up within a fundamentalist religion will receive early socialisation to practices such as prayer, the reading of holy texts, and singing, within their family and religious community. It is argued that the practice of prayer can be therapeutic as an individual practice or communal event (Kania, 2006, p. 112). As has become apparent, in comparison to growing up within Christianity, Muslims approach the religious training of children more intensely, with children attending Qur'an classes three times a week after school (Scourfield et al., 2017). While this stereotypical approach ignores diversity between group practices, the mainstream Sunni Muslim practice of adults praying five times a day and repeating passages of the Qur'an suggests religious commitment. This was seen as contributing to the intergenerational transmission of practices, exemplifying this way of life to young people and promoting close familial relationships, unity, and solidarity. This latter point is demonstrated in the marking of Shabbat[12] by Jews and

[12] The Friday night ritual of welcoming in the Sabbath.

the symbolism of Communion[13] to Christians. Religious rituals are integral to life for some Islamic families who dedicate every minute to their faith (Marks, 2004; Marks et al., 2017). The impact of religious practices on the stability of family relationships (Lambert & Dollahite, 2006; Lu et al., 2012) has been studied, with one qualitative study of 445 Christian, Jewish, and Muslim families identifying greater physical and mental health when family religious practices were regularly engaged with (Marks et al., 2012).

The declaration that regardless of religious association, 'all creatures make rituals for the sake of survival, order or comfort' (Anderson, 2010, p. 41) is not surprising, given that rites of passage rituals occur in relation to life events such as baptisms, christenings, weddings, funerals, memorials, burials, cremations, wakes, as significant changes of life circumstances are acknowledged (Shep Jeffreys, 2011). These make important contributions because they create good memories, which are vital for mental and physical health. One exception is research by Spagnola and Fiese (2007), which pinpointed some benefits for young people, including improved mental health, higher academic achievement, and improved social skills, although the rituals did not have to be religious ones. Conversely, some studies find that collective religious rituals might undermine parent–child relationships, especially if teenagers experienced the involvement as compulsory or boring (Strahan, 1994). Ahmed and Amer (2012) recognise that Islamic teenagers often need more independence during their identity-forming years, with others highlighting that family harmony can break down when young people move away from their parents' religious rituals and practices (Roer-Strier & Sands, 2001, 2004; Sands & Roer-Strier, 2004; Stokes & Regnerus, 2009). Rossano (2012) reveals that family routines and rituals not only bind family members together emotionally, but they are also the primary mechanisms by which cultural and religious values, beliefs, and traditions are passed from one generation to another. Although Saroglou's (2011, p. 1332) findings demonstrate that 'believing and belonging' are the strongest religious dimensions within orthodox groups, it has become obvious

[13] Communion is a practice meant to be observed by Christians.

that there has been very little focus on the effects on children in their developmental years, despite the potential impact on adult health.

References

Ahmed, S. & Amer, M. M. (2012). *Counselling Muslims. Handbook of mental health issues and interventions.* Taylor and Francis Group.
Anderson, H. (2010). How rituals heal. *World & World, 30*(1), 41–50.
Ashley, O. (2015). *The Bible, wisdom and human nature.* CWR.
Azarian, B. (2016). Apeirophobia: The fear of eternity. Which is scarier, death or everlasting life? *The Atlantic.* https://www.theatlantic.com/science/archive/2016/09/apeirophobia-the-fear-of-eternity/498368/
Bagher, G. B., Miner, M., & Proctor, M.-T. (2013). Attachment to God in Islamic spirituality. *Journal of Muslim Mental Health, 7*(2), 77–104. https://doi.org/10.3998/jmmh.10381607.0007.205
Bandura, A. (1977). *Social learning theory.* Prentice Hall.
Bartkowski, J. P., Xu, X., & Levin, M. L. (2008). Religion and child development: Evidence from the early childhood longitudinal study. *Social Science Research, 37*, 18–36. https://doi.org/10.1016/j.ssresearch.2007.02.001
Beck, R., & McDonald, A. (2004). Attachment to God: The attachment to God inventory, tests of working model correspondence, and an exploration of faith group differences. *Journal of Psychology and Theology, 32*(2), 92–103. https://doi.org/10.1177/009164710403200202
Berliner D., & Sarró, R. (2007). On learning religion. An introduction. In D. Berliner & R. Sarró (Eds.), *Learning religion: Anthropological approaches* (pp. 1–17). Berghahn.
Birtwistle, L., & Smith, L. (2012). *Children growing up with religion: Ten narratives explored.* York Publishing Services.
Bottoms, B. L., Shaver, P. R., Goodman, G. S., & Qin, J. (1995). In the name of God: A profile of religion-related child abuse. *Journal of Social Issues, 51*(2), 85–111. https://doi.org/10.1111/j.1540-4560.1995.tb01325.x
Bowlby, J. (1969). *Attachment and loss, volume 1: Attachment.* Basic Books.
Burr, W. R., Marks, L. D., & Day, R. D. (2012). *Sacred matters: Religion and spirituality in families.* Routledge.
Chen, Y., & VanderWeele, T. J. (2018). Associations of religious upbringing with subsequent health and wellbeing from adolescence to young adult: An

outcome-wide analysis. *American Journal of Epidemology, 187*(11), 2355–2364. https://doi.org/10.1093/aje/kwy142

De Sondy, A, Gonzalez, M. A., & Green, W. S. (2021). *Judaism, Christianity, and Islam. An introduction to monotheism.* Bloomsbury Academic.

Dollahite, D. C., Hawkins, A. J., & Parr, M. R. (2012). Something more: The meanings of marriage for religious couples in America. *Marriage & Family Review, 48*(4), 339–362.

Erikson, E. H. (1950). *Childhood and society*. Norton.

Frisk, L. (2018a). Growing up in controversial minority religions: Constructions of childhood. In L. Frisk„ S. Nilsson, & P. Akerback (Eds.), *Children in minority religions. Growing up in controversial religious groups* (pp. 64–94). Equinox.

Frisk, L. (2018b). Religion, parenting and child corporal punishment: The example of the Twelve Tribes. In L. Frisk, S. Nilsson, & P. Akerback (Eds.), *Children in minority religions. Growing-up in controversial religious groups* (pp. 208–230). Equinox.

Goodman, M. A., & Dollahite, D. C. (2006). How religious couples perceive the influence of God in their marriage. *Review of Religious Research, 48*, 141–155.

Goodman, M. A., Dollahite, D. C., Marks, L. D., & Layton, E. (2013). Religious faith and transformational processes in marriage. *Family Relations, 62*(5), 808–823. https://doi.org/10.1111/fare.12038

Gorsuch, R. L. (1968). The conceptualization of God as seen in adjective ratings. *Journal for the Scientific Study of Religion, 7*, 56–64. https://doi.org/10.2307/1385110

Granqvist, P. (2014). Mental health and religion from an attachment viewpoint: Overview with implications for future research. *Mental Health, Religion & Culture, 17*(8), 777–793. https://doi.org/10.1080/13674676.2014.908513

Green, A. A. (1905). The religious training of children among the Jews. In A. Strhn, S. G. Parker, & S. B. Ridgely (Eds.), *The Bloomsbury reader in religion and childhood* (pp. 161–163). Bloomsbury Academic.

Greenberg, D., & Witztum, E. (2001). *Sanity & sanctity: Mental health work among the Ultra-Orthodox in Jerusalem.* Yale University Press.

Hatch, T. G. (2015). *Mishpacha in the America Diaspora: An exploratory study of highly-involved Jewish families.* PhD thesis, Louisiana State University. http://digitalcommons.lsu.edu/gradschool_dissertations/519

Heimlich, J. (2011). *Breaking their will. Shedding light on religious child maltreatment*. Prometheus Books.

Holden, G., & Williamson, P. A. (2014). Religion and child well-being. In A. Ben-Arieh, F. Casas, I. FrØnes, & J. E. Korbin (Eds.), *Handbook of child well-being* (pp. 1137–1169). Springer Science. https://doi.org/10.1007/978-90-481-9063-8_158

Hood, R. W. Jr, Hill, P. C., & Spilka, B. (2018). *The psychology of religion: An empirical approach* (5th ed.). Guildford Press.

Horton, A. L., & Williamson, J. A. (1998). *Abuse and religion: When praying isn't enough.* Heath.

Houser, M. E., & Welch, R. D. (2013). Hope, religious behaviors, and attachment to God: A trinitarian perspective. *Journal of Psychology and Theology, 41*(4), 281–297. https://doi.org/10.1177/009164711304100402

Ineichen, B. (2019). Losing the rapture: Escaping from fundamentalist Christian belief. *Mental Health, Religion & Culture, 22*(7), 661–673. https://doi.org/10.1080/13674676.2018.1557872

Kania, W. (2006) Healthy religion: A psychological guide to a mature faith: Author House.

Kaufman, G. D. (1981). *The theological imagination: Constructing the concept of God.* Westminster Press.

Koenig, H. G., & Larson, D. B. (2001). Religion and mental health: Evidence for an association. *International Review of Psychiatry, 13*, 67–78. https://doi.org/10.1080/09540260124661

Ladd, K. L., McIntosh, D. N., & Spilkam, V. (1998). Children's God concepts: Influences of denomination, age, and gender. *International Journal for the Psychology of Religion, 8*, 49–56. https://doi.org/10.1207/s15327582ijpr0801_6

Lambert, N. M., & Dollahite, D. C. (2006). How religiosity helps couples prevent, resolve, and overcome marital conflict. *Family Relations, 55*, 439–449. https://doi.org/10.1111/j.1741-3729.2006.00413.x

Lees, J., & Horwath, J. (2009). Religious parents … just want the best for their kids: Young people's perspectives on the influence of religious beliefs on parenting. *Children and Society, 23*, 162–175. https://doi.org/10.1111/j.1099-0860.2008.00164.x

Lu, Y., Marks, L., & Apavaloiae, L. (2012). Chinese immigrant families and Christian faith community: A qualitative study. *Family and Consumer Sciences Research Journal, 41*, 118–130. https://doi.org/10.1111/fcsr.12002

Main, M. (1990). Cross-cultural studies of attachment organization: Recent studies, changing methodologies, and the concept of conditional strategies. *Human Development, 33*(1), 48–61.

Marich, J. (2024). *You lied to me about God.* North Atlantic Books.

Marks, L. (2004). Sacred practices in high religious families: Christian, Jewish, Mormon, and Muslim perspectives. *Family Process, 43*(2), 217–231. https://doi.org/10.1111/j.1545-5300.2004.04302007.x

Marks, L. D., Dollahite D. C., & Barker, K. (2012). Don't forget home. The importance of sacred rituals in families. In J. Hoffman (Ed.), *Understanding religious rituals* (pp. 186–203). Routledge.

Marks, L., Hatch, T. G., & Dollahite, D. C. (2017). Sacred practices and family processes in a Jewish context: Shabbat as the weekly family ritual par excellence. *Family Process, 57*(2), 448–461. https://doi.org/10.1111/famp.12286

McGrath, A. (2025). *Why we believe. Finding meaning in uncertain times.* Oneworld Publications.

Miller, A. (1987). *The drama of being a child: The search for the true self.* Virago Press.

Miner, M., Ghobary, B., Dowson, M., & Proctor, M.-T. (2014). Spiritual attachment in Islam and Christianity: Similarities and differences. *Mental Health, Religion & Culture, 17*(1), 79–93. https://doi.org/10.1080/13674676.2012.749452

Mohr, S., Brandt, P.-Y., Borras, L., Gillièron, C., & Huguelet, P. (2006). Towards an integration of spirituality and religiousness into the psychosocial dimension of schizophrenia. *The American Journal of Psychiatry, 163*(11), 1952–1959.

Okagaki, L., & Bevis, C. (1999). Transmission of religious values: Relations between parents' and daughters' beliefs. *The Journal of Genetic Psychology, 160*(3), 303–318. https://doi.org/10.1080/00221329909595401

Piaget, J. (1936). *Origins of intelligence in the child*. Routledge.

Roer-Strier, D., & Sands, R. G. (2001). The impact of religious intensification on family relations: A South African example. *Journal of Marriage and Family, 63*, 868–880. https://doi.org/10.1111/j.1741-3737.2001.00868.x

Roer-Strier, D., & Sands, R. G. (2004). Families challenged by religious change: A cross-cultural comparison of mothers' images of their daughters. *Families in Society, 85*, 485–594. https://doi.org/10.1177/104438940408500407

Rossano, M. J. (2012). The essential role of ritual in the transmission and reinforcement of social norms. *Psychological Bulletin, 138*(3), 529–549. https://doi.org/10.1037/a0027038

Sands, R. G., & Roer-Strier, D. (2004). Impact of religious difference and geographic distance on intergenerational family continuity. *Family Relations, 53*, 102–110. https://doi.org/10.1111/j.1741-3729.2004.00014.x

Saroglou, V. (2011). Believing, bonding, behaving, and belonging: The big four religious dimensions and cultural variation. *Journal of Cross-Cultural Psychology, 42*(8), 1320–1340. https://doi.org/10.1177/0022022111412267

Scourfield, J., Gilliat-Ray, S., Khan, A., & Otri, S. (2017). Learning to be a Muslim. In A. Strhn, S. G. Parker, & S. B. Ridgely (Eds.), *The Bloomsbury reader in religion and childhood* (pp. 123–130). Bloomsbury Academic.

Shep Jeffreys, J. (2011). *Helping grieving people—When tears are not enough. A handbook for care providers* (2nd ed.). Routledge.

Simonic, B., Mandelj, T. R., & Novsak, R. (2013). Religious-related abuse in the family. *Journal of Family Violence, 28*, 339–349. https://doi.org/10.1007/s10896-013-9508-y

Spagnola, M., & Fiese, B. H. (2007). Family routines and rituals: A context for development in the lives of young children. *Infants & Young Children, 20*(4), 284–299. https://doi.org/10.1097/01.IYC.0000290352.32170.5a

Steege, M. K. (2010). *The spirit-led life: A Christian encounter with internal family systems.* M. K. Steege.

Stokes, C. E., & Regnerus, M. D. (2009). When faith divides family: Religious discord and adolescent reports of parent-child relations. *Social Science Research, 38*(1), 155–167. https://doi.org/10.1016/j.ssresearch.2008.05.002

Stott, R. (2017), In the Days of Rain. A Daughter, A Father, A Cult. London: 4th Estate.

Strahan, B. J. (1994). *Parents, adolescents, and religion.* Avondale Academic Press.

Strhan, A. (2017). Children in contemporary british evangelicalism. In A. Strhan, S. G. Parker, & S. B. Ridgely (Eds.), *The Bloomsbury reader in religion and childhood* (pp. 51–60). Bloomsbury Academic.

US Legal Inc. (2019). *Religious upbringing law and legal definition.* https://definitions.uslegal.com/r/religious-upbringing/

Winell, M. (2020a). *Christianity and children.* https://journeyfree.org/article/christianity-and-children/

Winell, M. (2020b). *The challenge of leaving religion and becoming secular.* https://journeyfree.org/article/the-challenge-of-leaving-religion-and-becoming-secular/

Yip, A. K. T., Keenan, M., & Page, S. (2011). *Religion, youth and sexuality: Selected key findings from a multi-faith exploration.* University of Nottingham.

6
The 'Them and Us' Culture and Imposed 'All-or-Nothing' Rigid Rules

A 'Them and Us' Culture

An emergent theme in the literature was that children growing up within religious fundamentalism will be kept separate from society (Lam & Cohen, 2020; Moritz et al., 2018). This can positively influence well-being in the form of 'pride, loyalty and perceived superiority' with affirmation from those who hold the same beliefs (Frisk, 2018a, pp. 67–68; Moritz et al., 2018), but result in being an insider within fundamentalist religion but an outsider in the world (Frisk, 2018a, p. 69). Marich (2024, p. 4) posits that people often frame their devotion to a religion or spiritual practice as 'the proverbial, I've found the way, I'm better than you' weapon to fill them with a perceived sense of superiority'.

Eva recognised that separation was an integral part of her growing-up years:

> *... you were taken from the world, you were different. A bit like the Israelites who used to have a blue fringe at the bottom of their clothes.*

Francesca Alexandra succinctly summed this up:

G. Harvey, *Fundamentalist Religious Childhoods and Adult Mental Health and Wellbeing*, https://doi.org/10.1007/978-3-032-20140-9_6

... we were elite, proper Christians. People who didn't have the right values were dismissed ... so, we're the only ones that are saved, and it would be as far-reaching as different denominations of Christianity, so I remember the Church of England being frowned upon. They're not proper Christians, but we were called to be peculiar people.[1] *We were taught to love your neighbours as yourself, which is fine, but it's imbalanced. There needs to be loving yourself, not in a selfish manner, but in a self-care way, and that wasn't there.*

In addition, Holly spoke about the effect of separateness on friendships:

... and you're not part of it ('the world'), it is like the cult you're excluded from, that you don't actually have friends. You've actually lost all your friends, because your friendship group are only within the church.

Maya also spoke about the negative restrictions of disconnection.

You can't see your friends, friends are bad, you should never have friends. We are the only people that you need. God is the only person that you need. You should be praying five times a day. You should be going to the mosque, reading the Qur'an. Why don't you do those things? You have time to do all of those things. Why can't you do that? You can't go to an after-school club, you can't be in the school play, you need to be going to the mosque, and you should be praying, and you should be doing what you're supposed to be doing, which is being a good Muslim.

While the influence of insider–outsider positions on health remains under-researched, a young person is probably an insider within fundamentalist religion but alienated in the outside world (Frisk, 2018a). The confusion of this for Francesca Alexandra is clear.

I was feeling so different, confused by the world because I wasn't prepared for it, rather naïve, I didn't know how to protect myself, and I didn't belong so it just meant I could have been eaten alive by the world... I wasn't prepared ..., poor autonomy, naivety, poor skills in autonomous thinking, feeling like

[1] The term 'peculiar people' means being special and is derived from Titus 2:14 in the Christian Bible.

an alien in the world with no idea how the world worked or how to defend myself within it, how to relate to it, to people in it.

Anna recognised the narrowness of only being allowed to socialise with other children who went to the same church. Yet, Rupert spoke about going to his non-Christian friends' houses after school, so, for him, the 'them and us' culture was lessened.

Several participants mentioned the in-language used in their family and group, which added to the sense of belonging. Anna talked about the terms that scared her as a child:

... washing your sins in the blood of the Lamb, lost sheep, backslider, lost faith, lost soul, the devil has won ...

Eva spoke about the in-terms used in the JW group, including 'congregation servant', 'field service', and the extant prejudice in the hierarchical, patriarchal, homophobic group.

Religious Prejudice

Kania's (2006, p. 140) perspective that 'the more a child and adolescent is exposed to the outside world, the more tolerant and accepting they are' suggests that being isolated in a 'them and us' culture leads to greater prejudice. This term is defined as 'a judgement or opinion formed before the facts are known; a preconceived idea, favourable or, more usually, unfavourable' (yourdictionary.com, 2021). Yet, one study revealed lower levels of bias, less selfishness, more happiness, and greater uprightness compared to other Americans (Hood et al., 2005). However, the common perception of religious fundamentalism as prejudiced towards those outside the group persists. Biases towards those outside of their narrow 'tightly knit enclaves' (Whiteley et al., 2017, p. 278) support the idea that fundamentalist religious groups have in-group/out-group attitudes.

This is illustrated in one ultra-orthodox Jewish community, which has been portrayed as 'insulated, totalistic, highly structured and tightly bound' (Berger, 2015, p. 670) with dogmatic, ethnocentric, and homophobic attitudes (Altemeyer & Hunsberger, 2005). Activities are restricted, and there is very little, if any, involvement in the secular world (lannacone, 1994, cited in Nica, 2019, p. 544). Ex-JW participants in Frisk's (2018a, pp. 67–68) research stated that 'you should prefer the company of other JWs. People outside could be a bad influence' (participant Patrik, ex-JW). Also, 'I never had any friends. My parents decided that I would be ostracised and bullied, for God's sake, I should not mix with other people because I was a Witness: they could influence me in negative ways' (participant Therese, ex-JW).

Children growing up within a fundamentalist religion will be influenced by negative prejudices towards others, religious and non-religious. This is confirmed in the research of Lam and Cohen (2020), which examined the mindsets of five-and six-year-old Islamic children of Pakistani heritage in both the United Kingdom (UK) and Saudi Arabia (SA) regarding in-group/out-group (Muslims versus non-Muslims) stances. The findings showed that children growing up within religious environments are significantly influenced by adult prejudices, and it is not surprising that one quantitative, questionnaire-based study of 291 first-year students at a Canadian University learned that in-group bias bestows positive favouritism towards people with the same religious beliefs (Moritz et al., 2018). It also enables collective self-esteem and group identity to exist 'with special meanings understood only by members of the group' (Jenkinson, 2019, p. 63). This has been called 'religious tribalism', which is defined as 'the distinct presence of powerful kingship groups (that) share explicit theological world views' (Meades, 2019, p. 178) and are intolerant of difference and diversity. This tallies with one of the emergent themes in an interpretative phenomenological analysis (IPA), which explored lesbian, gay, bisexual, and transgender plus (LGBT+)[2] experiences within the Abrahamic traditions. 'Participants' experiences were of boundaries that demarcated what was allowed, who was accepted and who and what was not permitted' (Meades, 2019, p. 178), leading to outsider status for the LGBT+ population.

[2] LGBT+ refers to lesbian, gay, bisexual and transgender, and is often used to encompass any sexual orientation or gender identity that does not correspond to heterosexual norms.

Some writers have referred to this as doctrinal maltreatment (Childers, 2012; Foster et al., 2015; Greene, 2013; Lucies & Yick, 2007; Super & Jacobson, 2011). All of this preserves the integrity of 'the marble edifice' (Jenkinson, 2016, p. 226) and keeps members free from other views, beliefs, and lifestyles that are judged to be unacceptable (Zieman, 2018). While the literature demonstrates that belonging in a religious community can be positively beneficial, the challenges of being an outsider remain largely unexplored. The revelations of one intergroup analysis of religion and prejudice found that while it was most apparent in highly religious groups, bias is present throughout the religious continuum, although less perceptible at the more liberal end (Jackson & Hunsberger, 1999).

The Cruelty of the 'Them and Us' Culture for Those Who Leave

In Chapter 4, it became apparent that the sense of bonding and belonging found within fundamentalist religious groups can be completely lost when members question or become non-compliant, resulting in ejection from the group and rejection by those once thought to be their 'nearest and dearest'. This 'universal way of punishing non-compliance' (Harvey, 2020, p. 7) literally discards people (Lifton, 1989), with non-believers being ousted from a group, excluded, and ignored, and social ties severed (Gutgsell, 2017, p. 18). *All members are forced to comply with the shunning edict (*Zieman, 2018*) issued by the religious leaders.* This 'dispensing of existence' (Lifton, 1989, cited in Jenkinson, 2023, p.190) is the punishment for non-compliance (Harvey, 2020, p. 7) and this illustrates the harshness of the 'them and us' culture as described by Eva.

> *I'm very strong, resilient and it's all okay and I've got freedom, I'm building a new life, and I can say all of that, but the reality is, it's heart-breaking because I've lost everything and at my age of nearly 40 how do you rebuild your life … I've definitely had my moments this year, I've felt completely alone, and*

those feelings become overwhelming, and you think, do I actually feel a bit suicidal?

Eva was the only co-researcher to explicitly talk about shunning. Her account matches statements that recognise that being shunned is one of the worst experiences a person can have (Zieman, 2018, cited in Harvey, 2020) because of the psychological turmoil and emotional pain that ensue (Berger, 2015; Fazzino, 2014; Fenelon & Danielsen, 2016; lannaccone, 1994). Shunning can result in 'religious trauma syndrome' (Winell, 2016, p. 1), yet the only focus on it in the literature is in relation to the JWs (Frisk, 2018b, pp. 149–170).

Imposed 'All-or-Nothing' Rigid Rules

All of the co-researchers spoke about the rigid rules that were an integral part of their growing-up years. This is not surprising, given that the literature reveals that parents often look to religion to provide a moral framework for their offspring (Holden & Williamson, 2014). While Holly was convinced that having rules could facilitate certainty and safety for some young people, the rigidity of the rules was what participants spoke about in the research interviews. Eva said that there were many dictates, which Anna described as:

… a plethora of shoulds, oughts, and musts in place.

This aligns with Mathis-Rimes's (2018, pp. 27–28) view, stating that religion contains moralistic rules without heart, created by humans. This also resonates with Berger's (2015, p. 670) perspective of the way that life within ultra-orthodox Judaism is controlled by a mass of rigid rules. Although Rupert believed that the rules in his childhood were ameliorated by love, he also recognised that fundamentalist religious rules were rigidly inflexible and affected the whole of life, because there was a paucity of other viewpoints considered by those imposing them.

Most of the regulations were aimed at managing behaviour, and some were related to what members could not do. These included not being allowed to watch television, especially on Sundays, not having sex outside marriage, drinking alcohol, or swearing, with women wearing make-up being prohibited. Conversely, other rules were about what members should do. For example, saying grace before each meal, reading the Bible, praying every day, and regularly attending church, the synagogue, or the mosque. Within Christianity, fundamentalist religious groups did not allow women to wear trousers, but they had to put on hats, especially when men were present in the religious community. Eva explained that the JWs were especially strict on this and recounted how, when hats were not available, tea towels were grabbed so that women could still cover their heads when men were present in a meeting. Holly did mention some rules also, including being forced to wear smart clothes to church and not being allowed to watch television on Sundays, sex outside of marriage being banned, and divorce and remarriage condemned (in later life, she felt ostracised by fellow church members for being a divorced and remarried Christian). She eloquently recognised their rigidity:

> *... very definite with all-or-nothing rules, you know, like hats. My friends needed to not be opposed to my Christian faith.*

Francesca Alexandra told me that there were lots of 'all-or-nothing rules', as they were not allowed to listen to non-Christian music, watch television, or read books that were seen as 'worldly'. They were also not permitted to wear make-up, go to the cinema, or wear trousers as women, with credit cards and alcohol being strongly disapproved of.

> *I remember hearing some other Christian music and resisting the urge to tap my foot because it was at a Christian youth event, because it was sinful ... That's terrible, really just having to shut off the natural desire to tap my foot ... Dancing was demonic. Trendy music, even if Christian, was sinful.*

Independent thinking and questioning were also forbidden because they were regarded as the product of a sinful lack of faith. Attendance at church on Sundays was mandatory, and she described the humiliation she felt when walking to church or getting off the bus carrying her hat, with a non-trendy hairstyle, while wearing her best 'starchy' clothes, and being forced to sit upright in services. Some school activities were seen as sinful and not allowed, so the end-of-term discos were banned. Instead, she would be isolated with the JW children, as everyone else enjoyed a treat. It is clear then that some imperatives were concerned with young people not being allowed to participate in activities that were normal for other 'wordly' children. Growing up within the JWs meant that Eva was not allowed to celebrate Christmas or birthdays.

She also gave an account of the increased management of her behaviour during her teenage years when morality rules became more rigidly enforced. Her experience echoes the literature that shows that fundamentalist religion seeks to impose a moral code on young people. Sex is viewed as only allowable within a marital relationship (The Watchtower, 2011), and anything else is unbiblical (Chryssides, 2016), including homosexuality, which was viewed within the organisation as:

> *... abhorrent and worse than anything.*

Such suppression was regarded as necessary so that the 'sinful disposition' (Holden & Williamson, 2014, p. 1140) of the child was eradicated in pursuance of purity and holiness. The effects on the child of standing out as different are summarised in the following words of Francesca Alexandra:

> *... if our clothes were old-fashioned, if our hair was not trendy, if we looked dowdy, if we weren't whatever it was, then all of that ... was seen as a good thing.*

The cruel discomfort of this for a young person is obvious and strengthens the argument made by Mathis-Rimes (2018) about moralistic rules without heart, which synchronises with Hatch's (2015) perspective. The pressure of some of the Muslim rules about the religious training of children in the mandatory attendance of Qur'an classes (Scourfield et al., 2017, p. 124) and the requirement to pray five times a day are evident in Maya's account; she spoke about being forced to completely cover her body when in public. Non-compliance with the rules meant that disobedience was punished physically, including being hit with a bamboo stick. Yet, she rebelled against the rule-based rigidity by pretending to fall asleep at the madrassa,[3] which she described as:

> *... a real moment of strength for being in such a disempowered position anyway, as a child, and then to have all those extra layers of power and control was a huge weight, and I think falling asleep is almost like trying to get away from all of that. The weight and that pressure, so it was a convenient thing for me to do, and it was a way of empowering myself in a really disempowering environment.*

Maya shared that the rigid rules meant that she was incarcerated and not allowed to be outside with friends or go to their houses, to have a boyfriend, or to do normal things. She believed that her mother and other family members displayed misogynistic behaviours, which triggered violence, rooted in both religious and cultural beliefs. She stated that all religions are patriarchal and authoritarian, although she believed that men and women in her family had great power.

> *Asian women are generally very strong and authoritarian, but also submissive, and Asian men are also authoritarian, so it's unfortunate for the children because they grow up with two authoritarian parents.*

She said that in her experience of growing up in a Sunni Muslim family, there were many rule-based expectations.

> *... to choose certain job roles, to marry at a certain age.*

Maya recognised the powerlessness of being a child in such a rule-based, restrictive environment. It is evident that she did not always comply with the rigid rules and sometimes questioned them; however, the reply to her questions was always:

> *... because God says so, that's the way God wants it to be. You don't understand, you don't get it, because I wasn't in touch with God. What a way to dismiss a legitimate question and a legitimate argument!*

---

[3] The Arabic word for an educational institute.

While some of the participants explicitly talked about the controlling nature of the rigid all-or-nothing rules, it is apparent that not all of the participants were contained to that extent. For example, Holly mentioned some rules, but the main one that affected her was the restrictions around who she spent time with. Hannah only mentioned rules in connection with the ultra-orthodox Hasidic sects. Berger (2015, p. 670) notes that within ultra-Orthodox Judaism, a multitude of prescribed rules about every aspect of life are 'strictly enforced and monitored', and rabbis are deferred to if there is any problem with rule interpretation. Such suppression was seen as necessary, so that the 'sinful disposition' (Holden & Williamson, 2014, p. 1140) of the child was eradicated in pursuance of purity and holiness.

Francesca Alexandra talked about the controlling nature of these rigid all-or-nothing rules, and it is apparent that many of the co-researchers were restricted in similar controlling ways. This must be understood with caution, as not all participants were subjected to this extent of control. Holly, for example, hardly mentioned rules, apart from the implicit ones around who she spent time with.

A plethora of rigid rules in co-researchers' stories emerged, with Francesca Alexandra identifying that the control of rigid rules created approved behaviour because not complying would result in punishment. It is important to recognise, however, that although Maya's account of the punishment for flouting the inflexible rules states that life was:

> *... extremely violent at times ... I was constantly in the middle of a war zone*

This was not the experience of all co-researchers; there are still many unanswered questions on this topic. Hannah's quotation below highlights the importance of understanding religion as on a spectrum with the liberal/cultural expressions at one end and the strict fundamentalist forms at the other. The following quotation from this co-researcher helps understand the extent of the plethora of rigid rules at the strict religious end.

> *That's almost one extreme, people that aren't particularly practising and then I've got this other extreme where the practice is everything, so every movement*

in somebody's life is predicated on what their rule book sort of tells them, and of course in Judaism, there are rules upon layers of rules and if you're not sure about something and you're living in an ultra-orthodox world (less choice), you go to your rabbi and the rabbi will provide you with what they think is the way forward, their interpretation. So, I think I'm telling you that there are quite extreme levels of deferring to someone's opinion to keep the rules, as best they can, and I think that can feel very containing. But I think it can also be very anxiety-provoking.

In this section, the 'them and us' culture of fundamentalist religion, as well as the integral and strictly imposed rigid rules, have been explored. In the next chapter, power, control, and authoritarian fearmongering will be discussed in the context of the challenges of a fundamentalist religious upbringing and its effect on wellbeing in adulthood.

References

Altemeyer, B., & Hunsberger, B. (2005). Fundamentalism and authoritarianism. In R. F. Paloutzian & C. L. Park (Eds.), *Handbook of the psychology of religion and spirituality* (pp. 378–393). Guildford Press.

Berger, R. (2015). Challenges and coping strategies in leavening an ultra-Orthodox community. *Qualitative Social Work, 14*(5), 670–686. https://doi.org/10.1177/1473325014565147

Childers, M. (2012). Holy havoc: Chaplains as first responders in healing spiritual abuse. *Chaplaincy Today, 28*(2), 37–42. https://doi.org/10.1080/10999183.2012.10767460

Chryssides, G. D. (2016). *Jehovah's witnesses. Continuity and change*. Routledge.

Fazzino, L. L. (2014). Leaving the church behind: Applying a deconversion perspective to Evangelical exit narratives. *Journal of Contemporary Religion, 29*(2), 249–266. https://doi.org/10.1080/13537903.2014.903664

Fenelon, A., & Danielsen, S. (2016). Leaving my religion: Understanding the relationship between religious disaffiliation, health, and well-being. *Social Science Research, 57*, 49–62. https://doi.org/10.1016/j.ssresearch.2016.01.007

Foster, K. A., Bowland, S. E., & Vosler, A. N. (2015). All the pain along with all the joy: Spiritual resilience in lesbian and gay Christians. *American*

Journal of Community Psychology, 55, 191–201. https://doi.org/10.1007/s10464-015-9704-4

Frisk, L. (2018a), Growing up in controversial minority religions: Constructions of childhood. In L. Frisk, S. Nilsson & P. Akerback (Eds.), *Children in minority religions. Growing up in controversial religious groups* (pp. 64–94). Equinox.

Frisk, L. (2018b). Diana Baumrind's parenting styles: Examples of the Osho movement and Jehovah's witnesses. In L. Frisk, S. Nilsson & P. Akerback (Eds.), *Children in minority religions. Growing up in controversial religious groups* (pp. 149–170). Equinox.

Greene, B. G. (2013). The use and abuse of religious beliefs in dividing and conquering between socially marginalized groups: The same-sex marriage debate. *Psychology of Sexual Orientation and Gender Diversity, 1*, 35–44. https://doi.org/10.1037/0003-066X.64.8.698

Gutgsell, J. (2017). *A loving provision? How former Jehovah's Witnesses experience shunning.* Master's thesis, Vrije Universiteit Brussels, Brussels. https://saysorry.org/wp-content/uploads/2019/09/shunning-and-disfellowshipping-in-jehovahswitnesses-by-j-gutgsell.pdf

Harvey, G. (2020). Ostracism. *ICSA Today, 11*(3), 7–9.

Hatch, T. G. (2015). *Mishpacha in the America Diaspora: An exploratory study of highly-involved Jewish families.* PhD thesis, Louisiana State University. http://digitalcommons.lsu.edu/gradschool_dissertations/519

Holden, G., & Williamson, P. A. (2014). Religion and child well-being. In A. Ben-Arieh, F. Casas, I. FrØnes, & J. E. Korbin (Eds.), *Handbook of child well-being* (pp. 1137–1169). Springer Science. https://doi.org/10.1007/978-90-481-9063-8_158

Hood, R. W., Hill, P. C., & Williamson, W. P. (2005). *The psychology of religious fundamentalism.* Guildford Press.

lannaccone, L. R. (1994). Why strict churches are strong. *American Journal of Sociology, 99*(5), pp.1180–1211. https://doi.org/10.1086/230409

Jackson, L. M., & Hunsberger, B. (1999). An intergroup perspective on religion and prejudice. *Journal for the Scientific Study of Religion, 28*(4), 509–523. https://doi.org/10.2307/1387609

Jenkinson, G. (2016). *Freeing the authentic self: Phases of recovery and growth from an abusive cult experience.* PhD thesis, University of Nottingham. https//.www.eprints/Nottingham/ac.uk/25707/1/161202/GillianJenkinson/FinalThesis.USE.pdf

Jenkinson, G. (2019). *Post-cult counselling workbook. A guide for your recovery and growth.* Hope Valley Counselling.

Kania, W. (2006). *Healthy religion: A psychological guide to a mature faith.* Author House.

Lam, V. L., & Cohen, T. (2020). Attitudes toward and inferred beliefs for religious ingroup/outgroup members: Muslim children of Pakistani heritage in the United Kingdom and Saudi Arabia. *Mental Health, Religion and Culture, 23*(1), 38–53. https://doi.org/10.1080/13674676.2019.1705266

Lifton, R. J. (1989). *Thought reform and the psychology of totalism. A study of "brainwashing" in China.* The University of North Carolina Press.

Lucies, C., & Yick, A. (2007). Images of gay men's experiences with antigay abuse: Object relations theory reconceptualized. *Journal of Theory Construction and Testing, 11*(2), 55–62.

Marich, J. (2024). *You lied to me about God.* North Atlantic Books.

Mathis-Rimes, C. (2018). *Cruel sanctuary: A young woman's battle to escape from a fanatical religious sect.* Amazon.

Meades, P. C. (2019). *An exploration of six lesbian and gay people's experiences of organised religion (Christianity, Islam, and Judaism). and their implications for psychotherapy: An interpretative phenomenological analysis (IPA).* Doctoral thesis, University of Middlesex. https://www.repository.mdx.ac.uk

Moritz, S., Lasfar, I., Reininger, K. M., & Ohis, I. (2018). Fostering mutual understanding among Muslims and non-Muslims through counterstereotypical information: An educational versus metacognitive approach. *The International Journal for the Psychology of Religion, 28*, 103–120. https://doi.org/10.1080/10508619.2018.1431759

Nica, A. (2019). Exiters of religious fundamentalism: Reconstruction of social support and relationships related to well-being. *Mental Health, Religion & Culture, 22*(5), 543–556. https://doi.org/10.1080/13674676.2019.1636015

Scourfield, J., Gilliat-Ray, S., Khan, A., & Otri, S. (2017). Learning to be a Muslim. In A. Strhn, S. G. Parker, & S. B. Ridgely (Eds.), *The Bloomsbury reader in religion and childhood* (pp. 123–130). Bloomsbury Academic.

Super, J. T., & Jacobson, L. (2011). Religious abuse: Implications for counselling lesbian, gay, bisexual, and transgender individuals. *Journal of LGBT Issues in Counseling, 5*(3–4), 180–196. https://doi.org/10.1080/15538605.2011.632739

The Watchtower. (2011-02). https://www.jw.org/en/publications/magazines/wp20110201/moral-values-children/2

Whiteley, C., Coyle, A., & Gleeson, K. (2017). An idiographic analysis of women's accounts of living with mental health conditions in Haredi Jewish

communities. *Mental Health, Religion & Culture, 20*(3), 277–293. https://doi.org/10.1080/13674676.2017.1354820
Winell, M. (2016). *Religious Trauma Syndrome: BABCP*. https://www.babcp.com/Review/RTS.aspx
YourDictionary. (2021). https://www.yourdictionary.com/prejudice
Zieman, B. (2018) *Shunned: A survival guide.* Amazon.

7

Power, Control, and Authoritarian Fearmongering

Power and Control

One of the emergent themes from the seminal work of Oakley and Kinmond (2013, pp. 23–24) was power or 'the capacity to influence' (Scazzero, 2015, p. 242). A religious leader claiming to have a divine appointment can lead to exploitation. Oakley and Kinmond (2013, p. 16) articulate that whenever there is a power differential, the potential for abuse exists. Later, Oakley and Humphreys (2019, p. 42) recognise that coercion and control are 'hallmarks of spiritual abuse'.

Lagone (2021, p. 6) succinctly summarises such subtleties and the effects of the misuse of power and control.

> … when a human being sets himself or herself up as a kind of selfish 'god' in another person's life, treating that person as an object that must be manipulated to serve the 'god's' needs, agendas, and goals. Deception lies at the heart of all forms of spiritual abuse. Therefore, spiritually abused individuals often do not identify themselves as such. Instead, they tend to blame themselves.

G. Harvey, *Fundamentalist Religious Childhoods and Adult Mental Health and Wellbeing*, https://doi.org/10.1007/978-3-032-20140-9_7

Figure 7.1 shows the Duluth power and control wheel (Domestic Abuse Intervention Programs, 2025), with the circumstances present in male-to-female domestic abuse. Coercive control is expressed in threats, intimidation, minimising, denying, blaming, and the misuse of male privilege, accompanied by emotional and economic abuse, which can lead to physical and/or sexual violence. Children can also be used as pawns in the employed power and control tactics. The opportunity for the misuse of power and control of young people is much greater than in a couple relationship, however, and this will be explored further in the following sections.

Power and Control Within Hierarchical and Patriarchal Fundamentalist Religion

The religious power and control wheel, developed by Anderson (2023), illustrates that many of the power and control dynamics in domestic abuse, as shown by the Duluth diagrams (Domestic Abuse Intervention Programs, 2025), can also be present in strict religious settings. On the one hand, Oakley and Humphreys (2019, p. 119) recognise that 'using authority, responsibility, power and influence for good can be of huge benefit to the organisations, teams and groups we lead', yet leaders also have a need to belong, which can result in 'self-serving practices that can expedite harmful practices'. Roudkovski (2024) agrees that powerful positions can be abused within a religious system by one person or by a group of people. She provides examples of pastors in churches, elders and deacons, ministry leaders, or committee members who, if they are motivated by 'power and prestige rather than service and love' (p. 68), can misuse their positions. Each element of the power and control wheel (Fig. 7.1) can exist within fundamentalist religion including the loss of autonomy, isolation, minimising, denying, blaming, threats, accusations and intimidation, sexuality and gender defining, emotional and spiritual abuse, and economic control, manipulation and exploitation, enforced accountability, censorship of decision-making, the requirement of secrecy and silence, coercion to conform, control through sacred texts or teaching, and the requirement of obedience to the abuser. Isolation

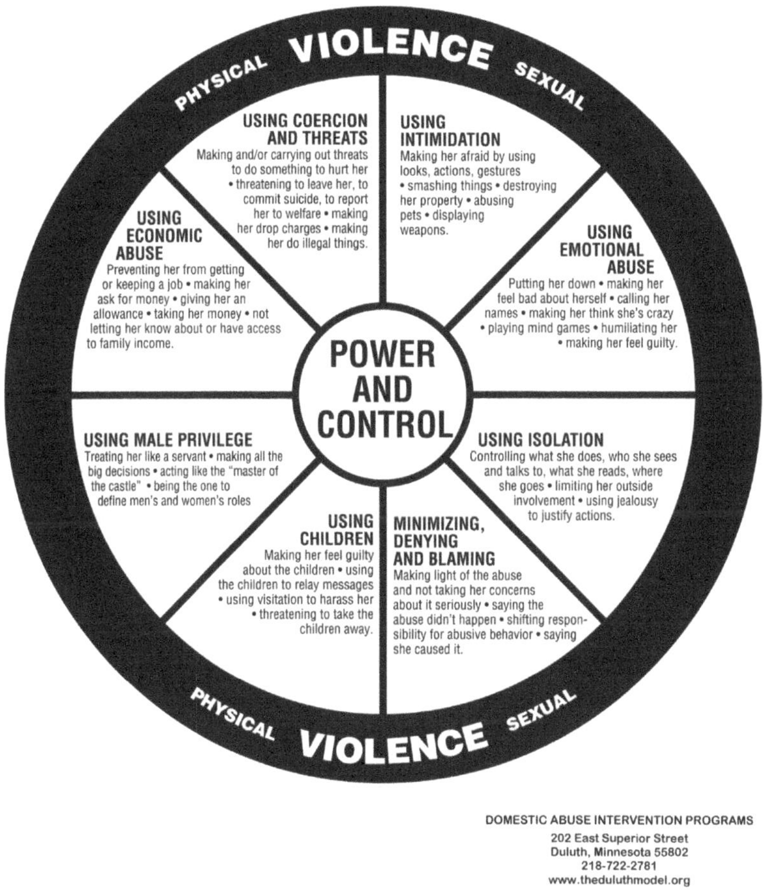

Fig. 7.1 Duluth power and control wheel (Domestic Abuse Intervention Programs, 2025)

can also be used as a form of control and a means of punishment, along with superiority and elitism. Harborne (2011, p. 2) insists that prayer can be directive and promote unhealthy dynamics when used manipulatively, especially if the person praying says that they have a word from God for the person being prayed for (Parsons, 2001).

Hannah was the one co-researcher who explicitly recognised the power and control that religious leaders have and stressed the importance of their authority not being misused.

> *… religion can be an absolute power, and I think one has to be very cautious as well of that … A rabbi has power and control, and it's about not misusing it and ensuring that power is not taken lightly.*

Yet, it is important to admit that religious leaders can be coercively controlled by other group members, although this is not often recognised in the literature. Swindle et al., (2024, p. 47) recognise that leaders can also be abused by 'the religious systems that employ them, being expected to be available at all times to support those who are ill, 'or in crisis', with unreasonable and contradictory expectations lacking clear boundaries leading to detrimental effects on their own personal relationships'. Pastors can also suffer vicarious trauma from listening to congregants as part of their work. Oakley and Humphreys' (2019, p. 9) assertion that coercive control can be 'top down from leadership' as well as from members is persuasive, as is their claim that 'spiritual abuse can happen to anyone and anyone can coerce and control another' (Oakley & Humphreys, 2019, p. 10).

High-demand religious groups have hierarchical and patriarchal systems that have historically elevated men to positions of power. For example, although there are a few women rabbis now, the majority remain male. Boys and men within the JWs have many more opportunities open to them than their female counterparts, and at the top of the organisational hierarchy, there are a few male leaders. Eva discussed her experiences related to gender within this group.

> *There was always the feeling that they (adult men) looked down on you and that you weren't good enough.*

Holly commented on the practical outworkings of the gender categorisations within the Baptist church that she grew up in:

> *… men had knowledge and women had feelings, which were less tangible.*

These accounts strengthen the assertion that women within fundamentalist religions are treated as inferior and have less power. Marich (2024, p. 10) gave the explanation that:

> Most, if not all, women have been spiritually abused in their lifetimes because of the patriarchal orientations of institutional religion and government control over women's lives.

This echoes with Swindle et al. (2024), who argue that women are especially susceptible to spiritual abuse, given the historic tradition of patriarchal, hierarchical systems resulting in limited opportunities for leadership or service. They posit that the 'submissive wives' theology within Christianity has sometimes pressurised women to stay in abusive and non-functional marriages because they are seen as the 'lesser gender', making them particularly vulnerable to religious abuse (pp. 44–45). Holly recalled that when she was going through a divorce, the blame for the breakup was placed entirely on her.

Power and Control Over Children Within Fundamentalist Religion

Research participants and therapy clients have all shared that, as children, they were powerless, the lowest in the hierarchy, with God at the top, the male leaders next, then women, and lastly children. Swindle et al., (2024, p. 24) convincingly state that children within strict religious communities are the most vulnerable to coercive control, given that they are already powerless, having been taught to be rule followers where obedience is mandatory, and asking questions and critical evaluation are forbidden. They highlight that caregivers often assume it is safe to leave children in church environments for extended periods, which may not be the case.

Some of the co-researchers also overtly recognised the powerlessness of children growing up within fundamentalist religion. Maya said this:

> *I was expected to be a Muslim like my family, with the ideologies being forced on me from a young age.*

Even Rupert acknowledged that he did not have a voice in the Baptist church he grew up in because children were expected to be respectful of adults.

The conclusion can only be that if being controlled is anxiety-provoking for adults, it is likely that, in their formative years, the powerlessness that children are subjected to must only increase the detrimental effects on them in later life. In line with this, writers such as Roudkovski (2024) and Swindle et al., (2024, p. 6) argue that some populations are more vulnerable to religious abuse than others. These include children, women, people of racial and ethnic minorities, those who identify as lesbian, gay, bisexual, transgender, queer+ (LGBTQ+), those who hold 'non-majority beliefs', and those who are deconstructing their religious beliefs.

Authoritarian Fearmongering Within Fundamentalist Religious Communities

Religious power and control are commonly increased by dogmatic teaching on subjects that can terrify children. Examples of this include being taught about hell, eternal damnation, being left behind at the second coming of Christ, the existence of jinns and demons, punishment for sin, the imminency of the end times, and Armageddon.

This was true for Anna, who was taught in a forced, controlling, and definite way.

> *I didn't even know there was a choice; it simply was, and it never crossed my mind to think any differently, and the spirit of criticality was certainly not supported, a sense of autonomy was certainly not encouraged, or criticality or decision-making or taking personal responsibility – instead, there was encouragement to pray about it.*

She felt that she was not in charge of her own destiny because she was always waiting to know God's will, or for the divine to reveal something which scared her. She now recognises this as coercively controlled fearmongering.

> *Hell wasn't a metaphor. There wasn't a plan B … that was part of the fear … You were entirely lost or entirely precious … These were the two polarities growing up, and there wasn't even purgatory (the middle ground).*

She also said that she believed that she was being constantly watched by God because she learned that he was omnipresent. The detrimental effects on her were obvious.

> *Being constantly scared was unhelpful to fitting in at school, and I felt on the outside looking in, although I wanted to belong.*

This correlates with Heimlich's (2011) argument that one form of religious maltreatment is scaring children with religious teachings such as spending eternity in hell, the existence of devils and demons, and God being portrayed as vindictive.

Francesca Alexandra also spoke about the effects of the extensive power and control that she faced, especially as, again, independent thinking and questioning were not allowed because they were viewed as disrespectful. She became wary of everyone as a result.

> *Don't think, don't question … as well as a lack of respect for authority, it also meant that having your own mind was sinful, it was a lack of faith, it was condemned. I couldn't breathe with homework. I couldn't breathe with friends outside the church. They might be the anti-Christ*[1] *anyway, so you'd better not go near them.*

---

[1] In some Christian teachings, this is a personal opponent of Christ expected to appear before the end of the world (Collins English Dictionary, 2021).

Authoritarian Fearmongering Within Fundamentalist Religious Families

> Abuse within families is behaviorally nuanced and emotionally complex. Always, it is within a dynamic of power and control that emotional and physical abuse is perpetuated. Abuse may manifest as physical (throwing, shoving, grabbing, blocking pathways, slapping, hitting, scratches, bruises, burns, cuts wounds, broken bones, fractures, damage to organs, permanent injury, or even murder), sexual (suggestive flirtatiousness, propositioning, undesired or inappropriate holding, kissing, fondling of sexual parts, oral sex, or any kind of forceful sexual activity), or emotional (neglect, harassment, shaming, threatening, malicious tricks, blackmail, unfair punishments, cruel or degrading tasks, confinement, abandonment). (Terkeurst, 2020, p. 249)

Religious abuse is not contained within communities, however, but also commonly occurs in fundamentalist religious families. Francesca Alexandra shared that her mother's mental health challenges facilitated the inequitable dynamics of power and control in childhood and later:

> *… so not allowed a voice. We couldn't question. Mum was an issue; I was aware of her power over me as a child and as an adult … That determined every action of mine, from getting the right help, from living well, from parenting my children, from marriage, it's pervasive in every aspect until I managed to get some healing.*

The child-rearing practices of religious fundamentalist parents are frequently driven by the teachings of religious leaders based on the holy texts and rooted in beliefs about children. It has become clear that authoritarian parenting (Baumrind, 1966, 1968), 'in which obedience is important and critical thinking is discouraged' (SOU, 1998, cited in Frisk, 2018b, p. 149), is evident in some of the participant accounts. For instance, Francesca Alexandra described 'religious child maltreatment' (Heimlich, 2011, p. 29) as scripture was 'rammed down her throat' at home by her mother as punishment for non-compliance, with such reprimands creating great fear so that she constantly lived in hyper-arousal.[2]

The authority that fundamentalist religious parents have over their children is undoubtedly detrimental and impactful, with identity formation being prescribed. Marich (2024, p. 32) expressed the extent of the control that she felt.

> When I was growing up, it didn't even cross my mind to be myself at school, especially because it was a Catholic school … that's how tight the chains of control remained on my developing personhood.

Winell (2020) asserts persuasively that Christian teaching around the self being bad and in need of salvation can negatively impact a child's formation, resulting in low self-worth and difficulties with decision-making. This resonates with Anna's account of being 'constantly scared', because of teaching around a literal belief in sin, the second coming of Christ, being left behind, and going to a real place called hell, as well as emotive words in hymns. She recalled the shame and guilt that she carried, which led to the repeated writing of confessionals and becoming 'a good girl' because that gained approval. She told me that she still struggles with decision-making.

Growing up in a fundamentalist Muslim family meant that Maya, too, was the victim of authoritarian fearmongering, and she spoke about the powerlessness she felt and the complete lack of choice she had as a child. These experiences add weight to concerns about parents 'beat(ing) their children into submission with religious clubs' (Carlson, 1995, p. 90), although this damaging behaviour is not limited to white Protestant households, which is where the literature focuses. So tough was the Sunni Muslim home environment in which Maya grew up that authoritarian fearmongering involved incidents of traumatising domestic violence, including a male relative breaking down her bedroom door when she refused to attend the mosque. Given the amount of domestic violence that happened, it is not surprising that the co-researcher described her childhood as:

---

[2] Hyper-arousal means to be constantly hyper-alert, ready for the next threat to occur.

> *... the black hole, an abyss of trauma, as I was constantly in the middle of a war zone.*

Her mother would shut down any 'free behaviour' by her siblings and herself, because of a terror of the bad jinns (demons) and the devil coming into the household. At one point, Maya asked her mother why she put God before her children, and the reply was that she was fearful of facing God on judgement day, and of being punished and sent to hell because her children were not Muslims. Yet, in Maya's words:

> *... I was often vocal and often standing up for myself and others, saying no, I'm not doing this, no, I'm not going to wear a scarf, no, I'm not going to the mosque, no, it's not ok to treat others like that and I was always met with a lot of extreme violence and backlash for that.*

Francesca Alexandra also spoke about the lack of power and control in her childhood, and the confusion of her mother being sometimes loving and caring, and very manipulative at other times. She said that her mother's mental health challenges enabled the inequitable dynamics of power and control, which have detrimentally impacted the mother-daughter relationship in the long term.

She movingly recalled her embarrassment at being forced to march up and down the street with a billboard around her neck, shouting end-times rhetoric. Despite this, Francesca Alexandra formed a secure bond with God. This adds substance to the perspective that God can become a religious child's attachment figure (Granqvist, 2014, pp. 777–780; Kaufman, 1981, p. 67), although this is dependent on a positive view of God rather than a powerful, angry, and punishing deity (Bagher et al., 2013; Heimlich, 2011; Miner et al., 2014). The picture that emerges is of parents having great power and control, with the influence of religious leaders barely mentioned in these texts.

Marich (2024) raises concerns about how young people would be treated if they refused to follow their caregivers' religion. She contends that 'parents often do not know what is best for their children's mental health and development, especially if the extremism of their religious belief prevents them from seeing their children as they are' (Marich, 2024, p. 31).

Some authors are concerned about children suffering neglect and emotional abuse, facilitated by parental religious world views (Bottoms et al., 1995; Simonic et al., 2013) and attitudes towards their offspring, world views are elevated by the disciplinary techniques used in some religious families (Bartkowski et al., 2008; Carlson, 1995) which can cause damage to the psyche (Cornah, 2006).

Marich (2024, pp. 30–31) perceptively sums up the lack of power and control that children often face in fundamentalist religious communities and families.

> As I see it now, any child under the legal age of adulthood in any culture can never fully make a decision freely if it feels that love and acceptance, not to mention a place to live and eat, is contingent on doing what your parents expect of you …

Figure 7.2 contains the Duluth equality wheel (Domestic Abuse Intervention Programs, 2025), which illustrates the features that are present in positive male–female strong domestic interactions. These include the polarised opposite aspects of negotiation, fairness, respect, trust, support, honesty, accountability, shared responsibility, economic partnership, and responsible parenting, which contrast sharply with the unhealthy dynamics demonstrated in Fig. 7.1. While this equality wheel is especially concerned with the healthy elements of male-to-female interactions, it can also be more broadly applied to other relationships and organisations and suggests that, when present, children are less likely to experience Adverse Religious Experiences (AREs).

The Duluth nurturing children wheel (Domestic Abuse Intervention Programs, 2025), shown in Fig. 7.3, illustrates the conditions that many children outside of high-demand religions grow up with. The healthy dynamics presented include the promotion of emotional and physical security, the giving of affirmation, encouragement and support, honouring autonomy while giving time and affection, trusting, and respecting children while also enabling them to self-care. This summarises Hannah's childhood in liberal, cultural Judaism.

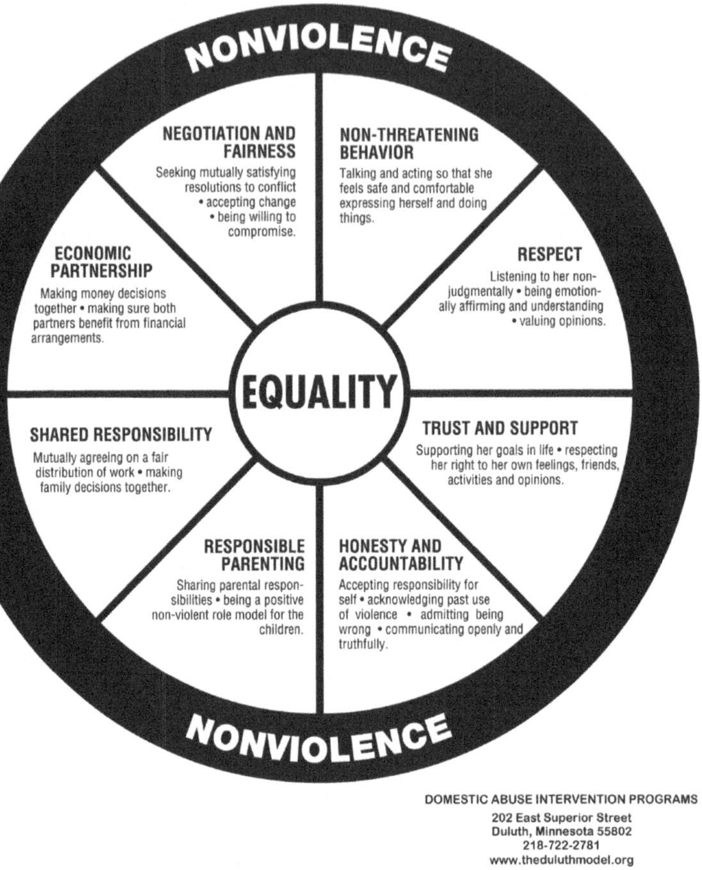

Fig. 7.2 Duluth equality wheel (Domestic Abuse Intervention Programs, 2025)

> *I was brought up in a very independent way… and had a Jewish education for my primary years, although not for secondary school … I was very immersed in Judaism from a very early age … e.g. Shabbat meals, so every weekend the meals were absolutely sacred and still are now. I grew up in a pretty practising Jewish home e.g. welcoming the Shabbat through the lighting of candles, usually by the woman in the household, but I was never made to feel that I'd be punished for keeping Shabbat or not, I think my parents would have been highly disappointed and I would have felt enormously guilty, but at the end of the day it was my own decision and the same is true for the next*

generation, my children, I'd rather they felt they'd come to their own decisions for the right reasons than to keep something for the sake of keeping it because then that would veer into the idea of abuse.

Consequently, it is not surprising that at the time of the research interviews, she radiated good health and wellbeing, compared to some of the

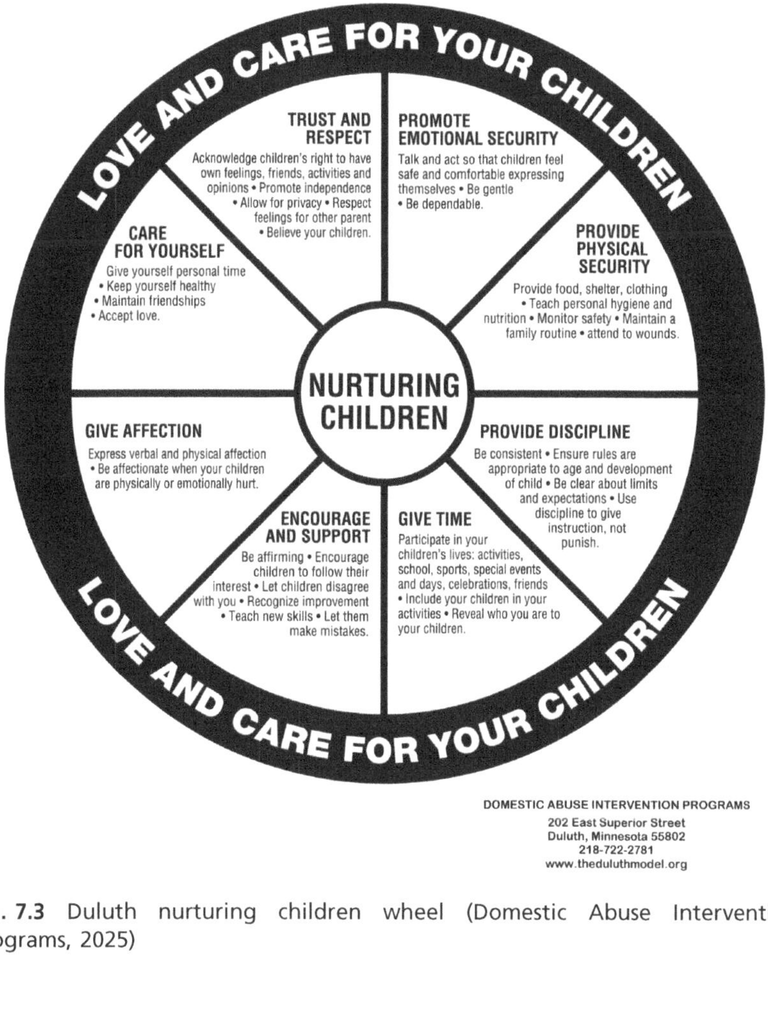
LOVE AND CARE FOR YOUR CHILDREN
TRUST AND RESPECT
Acknowledge children's right to have own feelings, friends, activities and opinions • Promote independence • Allow for privacy • Respect feelings for other parent • Believe your children.
PROMOTE EMOTIONAL SECURITY
Talk and act so that children feel safe and comfortable expressing themselves • Be gentle • Be dependable.
CARE FOR YOURSELF
Give yourself personal time • Keep yourself healthy • Maintain friendships • Accept love.
PROVIDE PHYSICAL SECURITY
Provide food, shelter, clothing • Teach personal hygiene and nutrition • Monitor safety • Maintain a family routine • attend to wounds.
NURTURING CHILDREN
GIVE AFFECTION
Express verbal and physical affection • Be affectionate when your children are physically or emotionally hurt.
PROVIDE DISCIPLINE
Be consistent • Ensure rules are appropriate to age and development of child • Be clear about limits and expectations • Use discipline to give instruction, not punish.
ENCOURAGE AND SUPPORT
Be affirming • Encourage children to follow their interest • Let children disagree with you • Recognize improvement • Teach new skills • Let them make mistakes.
GIVE TIME
Participate in your children's lives: activities, school, sports, special events and days, celebrations, friends • Include your children in your activities • Reveal who you are to your children.
LOVE AND CARE FOR YOUR CHILDREN
DOMESTIC ABUSE INTERVENTION PROGRAMS
202 East Superior Street
Duluth, Minnesota 55802
218-722-2781
www.theduluthmodel.org

Fig. 7.3 Duluth nurturing children wheel (Domestic Abuse Intervention Programs, 2025)

other participants who have had health challenges throughout their adult lives.

In reality, all of the other co-researchers recognised the lack of control and choice open to them as disempowered children being trained to be obedient. As is evident in Fig. 7.4, the Duluth abuse of children wheel (Domestic Abuse Intervention Programs, 2025), there are many common denominators between the general exploitation of young people and the religious abuse of minors. As can be seen, contributory factors include intimidation, using institutions to threaten punishment from God, isolation from peers or grandparents, emotional abuse such as shaming, put-downs, and/or name-calling, economic abuse, for example, using money to control behaviour, making threats, using adult privilege, and instilling fear through intimidation. Some ways of controlling behaviour by physical punishment are outlined on the rim of the wheel, and these include committing incest, sexual touching and kissing, the sexualisation of children's behaviour, and violent physical punishments such as pinching, hitting, kicking, pushing, twisting arms, and choking. This resonates with the literature, which emphasises that emotional abuse is often accompanied by neglect from powerful caregivers, facilitated by parental beliefs about children and their religious convictions (Bottoms et al., 1995, p. 85). As has become apparent, concerns have been raised about the corrective strategies used in some religious households, mainly conservative Protestant families (Bartkowski et al., 2008), with scripture being used to justify the physical and sexual abuse of children (Horton & Williamson, 1998). This synchronises with Frisk's (2018a, 2018b, 2018c) assertion that some people argue that the Bible supports the physical disciplining of children for correction purposes. An example is provided of the Twelve Tribes (a controversial religious movement within Christianity), who discipline children by using a little stick to spank young children. Clearly, young children, such as Maya, are completely powerless against those whose role is protection but who instead misuse adult privilege, threats, and intimidation to coercively control behaviour.

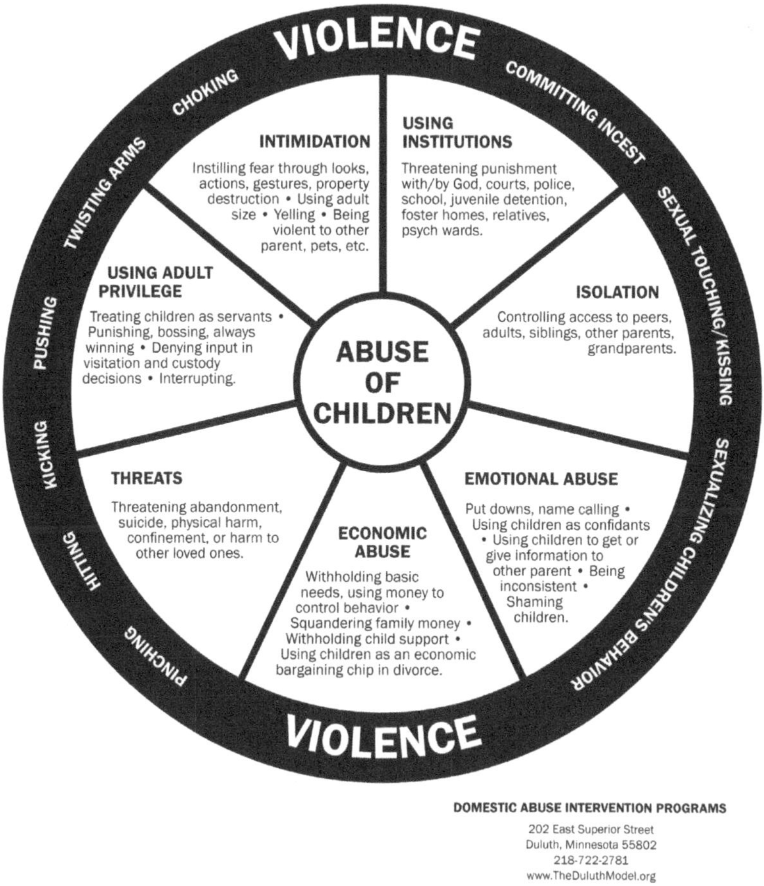
VIOLENCE
CHOKING
COMMITTING INCEST
TWISTING ARMS
SEXUAL TOUCHING/KISSING
PUSHING
KICKING
SEXUALIZING CHILDREN'S BEHAVIOR
HITTING
PINCHING
VIOLENCE
INTIMIDATION
Instilling fear through looks, actions, gestures, property destruction • Using adult size • Yelling • Being violent to other parent, pets, etc.
USING INSTITUTIONS
Threatening punishment with/by God, courts, police, school, juvenile detention, foster homes, relatives, psych wards.
USING ADULT PRIVILEGE
Treating children as servants • Punishing, bossing, always winning • Denying input in visitation and custody decisions • Interrupting.
ISOLATION
Controlling access to peers, adults, siblings, other parents, grandparents.
ABUSE OF CHILDREN
THREATS
Threatening abandonment, suicide, physical harm, confinement, or harm to other loved ones.
EMOTIONAL ABUSE
Put downs, name calling • Using children as confidants • Using children to get or give information to other parent • Being inconsistent • Shaming children.
ECONOMIC ABUSE
Withholding basic needs, using money to control behavior • Squandering family money • Withholding child support • Using children as an economic bargaining chip in divorce.
DOMESTIC ABUSE INTERVENTION PROGRAMS
202 East Superior Street
Duluth, Minnesota 55802
218-722-2781
www.TheDuluthModel.org

Fig. 7.4 Duluth abuse of children wheel (Domestic Abuse Intervention Programs, 2025)

The Ethics of Influencing and Safeguarding Children

Safeguarding children has always been critically important, but never as imperative as in the current national and global climate. However, it is acknowledged that at the time of the author's and co-researchers' childhoods, very little attention was given to the protection of minors. Yet, it is surprising that it was only in 2021 that the update of the UK Domestic Abuse Act included spiritual abuse for the first time. The global aspects of religion namely 'believing, bonding, behaving and belonging' (Saroglou, 2011, p. 1320), alternatively conceptualised as 'religious community, religious beliefs, and religious practices' (Hatch, 2015, p. 38), enable an understanding of the ethics of influence alongside the potential benefits for children of growing up in a strict religious environment. What has become apparent is that very little research has focused on the developmental experiences of children in strict religious contexts. This is a crucial area of missing information, because while religion is only one part of child development (Birtwistle & Smith, 2012, p. 1), it is a central one.

Controversially, Tillson (2019, p. 39) maintains that while children need to be protected from harm, they do not have the 'right to self-determination' because they are not yet adults. Despite the lack of research, the United Nations Convention states that all children have rights regardless of ethnicity, gender, religion, first language, ability, or any other factor (UNICEF, 2021). Some religious parents regard child-rearing as a sacred responsibility, although the tension that religious parents hold between their right to pass on their own beliefs and values and their avoidance of indoctrination[3] (Hand, 2002) is transparently obvious. While parents arguably have a moral right to share their religion with their children, this potentially infringes on the child's entitlement to have an unbiased future, especially if narrow religious beliefs and practices (Morgan, 2005) develop. These arguments fail to acknowledge that parents have their own belief systems about parenting and follow their guidelines about child-rearing to differing degrees (Frisk, 2018a). Consequently, the impact on each child will vary. In the context of faith schools, Worsley (2008, p. 76) argues that indoctrination breaches the United Nations conventions clauses to protect the 'rights of the child', especially when other worldviews are withheld.

It is imperative to recognise that while fundamentalism can provide secure bulwarks in an ever-changing, chaotic world, it is crucial to protect children and young people from the power, control, and authoritarian fearmongering of high-demand religion. There can be little doubt that

[3] Indoctrination is teaching someone to accept a set of beliefs without questioning.

some parents are convinced that while their young people live under the same roof, they are expected to go to the same church, mosque, or synagogue. Tenants of reproductive justice maintain that parents can raise their children in whatever way they feel is safe and sustainable for all involved. The remaining question, however, is whether they are creating safe home and communal environments where the young person can ask questions and express their doubts about the way they are being raised, where they are nurtured and valued for who they are, and can develop their authentic identity. After all, religious abuse is multilayered, permeating communities and families with potentially devastating effects in adult life, as encapsulated in the following quotation.

> Spiritual abuse is a misuse of power in a spiritual context whereby spiritual authority is distorted to the detriment of those under its leadership. It is a multifaceted and multilayered experience that includes acts of commission and omission, aimed at producing conformity. It is both process and event, influencing one's inner and outer worlds, and has the potential to affect the biological, psychological, social and spiritual domains of the individual. (Ward, 2011, p. 913)

While more research into the long-term effects of children being coercively controlled is needed, Oakley and Humphreys (2019) argue that rather than engage in the customary debates about whether a group is a cult or not, the focus needs to be on the behaviour of those in authority, because although religious abuse is more likely at the strictly religious end of the continuum with safe behaviour at the other, many inappropriate actions fit in between the two extremities.

In summary, it is important to note that some participants in the research study did not experience manipulative power and control and authoritarian fearmongering to the same extent as others. This resonates with one literature review that found that studies of religious manipulation in the family setting are rare (Simonic et al., 2013). This is evident in the accounts of Holly, Hannah, and Rupert, who all spoke warmly about their family and their heritage of religious practices and attendance at their religious community. They also talked about the value of learning about religious matters from a young age, with habits, both cultural and religious, continuing throughout their adult life to the present day and on to future generations. Rupert experienced secure family and church belonging and also has had a positive God-image, enabling a secure base with the divine throughout his life. This is an important recognition because a child's feeling makes possible the creation of a protective base and safe haven, enabling a healthy nervous system to regulate distress (Gerhardt, 2015; Rholes & Simpson, 2004), which opens up the possibility of good health in the future. The opposite is sadly true for those who experience abusive power and control from religious families and communities in their formative years, whose nervous system is less likely to be regulated and who may suffer greater health challenges in adulthood. The impact on adult mental health, physical wellbeing, and spirituality will be discussed in Chapter 8.

References

Anderson, L. E. (2023). *When religion hurts you. Healing from religious trauma and the impact of high-control religion.* Brazos Press.

Bagher, G. B., Miner, M., & Proctor, M.-T. (2013). Attachment to God in Islamic spirituality. *Journal of Muslim Mental Health, 7*(2), 77–104. https://doi.org/10.3998/jmmh.10381607.0007.205

Bartkowski, J. P., Xu, X., & Levin, M. L. (2008). Religion and child development: Evidence from the Early Childhood Longitudinal Study. *Social Science Research, 37*, 18–36. https://doi.org/10.1016/j.ssresearch.2007.02.001

Baumrind, D. (1966). Effects of authoritative parental control on child development. *Child Development, 37*(4), 887–907. https://doi.org/10.2307/1126611

Baumrind, D. (1968). Authoritarian vs authoritative parental control. *Adolescence, 3*, 252–272.

Birtwistle, L., & Smith, L. (2012). *Children growing up with religion: Ten narratives explored.* York Publishing Services.

Bottoms, B. L., Shaver, P. R., Goodman, G. S., & Qin, J. (1995). In the name of God: A profile of religion-related child abuse. *Journal of Social Issues, 51*(2), 85–111. https://doi.org/10.1111/j.1540-4560.1995.tb01325.x

Carlson, W. (1995). *Why do Christians shoot their wounded?* Authentic Lifestyle Publications/Media.

Collins English (2021). https://www.collinsdictionary.com/dictionary/english

Cornah, D. (2006). *The impact of spirituality on mental health.* Mental Health Foundation.

Domestic Abuse Intervention Programs. (2025). https://www.TheDuluthModel.org

Frisk, L. (2018a). Growing up in controversial minority religions: Constructions of childhood. In L. Frisk, S. Nilsson, & P. Akerback (Eds.), *Children in minority religions. Growing up in controversial religious groups* (pp. 64–94). Equinox.

Frisk, L. (2018b). Diana Baumrind's parenting styles: Examples of the Osho movement and Jehovah's Witnesses. In L. Frisk, S. Nilsson, & P. Akerback (Eds.), *Children in minority religions. Growing up in controversial religious groups* (pp. 149–170). Equinox.

Frisk, L. (2018c). Religion, parenting and child corporal punishment: The example of the Twelve Tribes. In L. Frisk, S. Nilsson, & P. Akerback (Eds.), *Children in minority religions. Growing up in controversial religious groups* (pp. 208–230). Equinox.

Gerhardt, S. (2015). *Why love matters. How affection shapes a baby's brain.* Routledge.

Granqvist, P. (2014). Mental health and religion from an attachment viewpoint: Overview with implications for future research. *Mental Health, Religion & Culture, 17*(8), 777–793. https://doi.org/10.1080/13674676.2014.908513

Hand, M. (2002). Religious upbringing considered. *Journal of Philosophy of Education., 3*(4), 545–557.

Harborne, L. (2011). *Working with issues of spirituality, faith, religion or belief.* BACP.

Hatch, T. G. (2015). *Mishpacha in the America Diaspora: An exploratory study of highly-involved Jewish families.* PhD thesis, Louisiana State University. http://digitalcommons.lsu.edu/gradschool_dissertations/519

Heimlich, J. (2011). *Breaking their will.* Prometheus Books.

Horton, A. L., & Williamson, J. A. (1998). *Abuse and religion: When praying isn't enough.* Heath.

Kaufman, G. D. (1981). *The theological imagination: Constructing the concept of God.* The Westminster Press.

Lagone, M. (2021). Guidelines for spiritually abused persons. In N. Damgaard (Ed.), *Wounded faith: Understanding and healing from spiritual abuse*. International Cultic Studies Association.

Marich, J. (2024). *You lied to me about God*. North Atlantic Books.

Miner, M., Ghobary, B., Dowson, M., & Proctor, M.-T. (2014). Spiritual attachment in Islam and Christianity: Similarities and differences. *Mental Health, Religion & Culture, 17*(1), 79–93. https://doi.org/10.1080/13674676.2012.749452

Morgan, J. (2005). Religious upbringing, religious diversity, and the child's right to an open future. *Studies in Philosophy and Education, 24*, 367–387.

Oakley, L., & Humphreys, J. (2019). *Escaping the maze of spiritual abuse*. Society for Promoting Christian Knowledge.

Oakley, L., & Kinmond, K. (2013). *Breaking the silence on spiritual abuse*. Palgrave Macmillan.

Parsons, S. (2001). *Ungodly Fear: Fundamentalist Christianity and the Abuse of Power*. Lion Books.

Rholes, W. S., & Simpson, J. A. (2004). *Attachment theory and religiosity: A summary of empirical research with implications for counselling Christian clients*. Guilford Publications.

Roudkovski, K. (2024). *Understanding spiritual abuse. What it is and how to respond*. B&H Academic.

Saroglou, V. (2011). Believing Bonding Behaving and Belonging. *Journal of Cross-Cultural Psychology, 42*(8), 1320–1340. https://doi.org/10.1177/0022022111412267

Scazzero, P. (2015). *The emotionally healthy leader*. Zondervan.

Simonic, B., Mandelj, T. R., & Novsak, R. (2013). Religious-related abuse in the family. *Journal of Family Violence, 28*, 339–349. https://doi.org/10.1007/s10896-013-9508-y

Swindle, P. J., Cashwell, C., & Tangen, J. L. (2024). *Counseling survivors of religious abuse*. Routledge.

Terkeurst, L. (2020). *Forgiving what you can't forget. Discover how to move on, make peace with painful memories, and create a life that's beautiful again*. Nelson Books.

Tillson, J. (2019). *Children, religion, and the ethics of influence*. Bloomsbury Academic.

UNICEF. (2021). *A summary of the UN Convention on the Rights of the Child*. https://www.unicef.org.uk/what-we-do/un-convention-child-rights/

Ward, D. J. (2011). The lived experience of spiritual abuse. *Mental Health, Religion & Culture, 14*(9), 899–915. https://doi.org/10.1080/13674676.2010.536206

Winell, M. (2020). *The challenge of leaving religion and becoming secular.* https://journeyfree.org/article/the-challenge-of-leaving-religion-and-becoming-secular/

Worsley, H. (2008). Church of England schools as centres for religious abuse or avenues for religious nurture? (The rights of children to encounter faith in the school context). *International Journal of Children's Spirituality, 13*(1), 75–83.

8

The Impact on Mental Health, Wellbeing, and Spirituality in Adulthood

Consideration of the adult experiences of the many people who grew up in strict religious environments is essential. Some will have had a happy childhood, bonded with caregivers who cherished them, and made a secure connection to a divine figure. Others will have found belonging in their church, mosque, hall, or synagogue, enjoyed fun and laughter, made friends with peers, and developed healthy connections. Pertinently, though, one author raises important questions about those whose experiences differed, as demonstrated in the quotation below:

> But what happens to those who are born into such fringe or even revolutionary lifestyles? They haven't chosen this life; will they grow up to wear it with pride and weather the criticism? Will they carry the same stigma? Will they be brainwashed? Can children be brainwashed, or are they just socialized in a different culture? (van Eck Duymaer van Twist, 2015, p. 3)

The findings of the Interpretative Phenomenological Analysis (Smith et al., 2009) research (Harvey, 2017), which examined Christian counsellors' lived experiences of the impact of spirituality when bereavement is the presenting issue, reveal that the mystery surrounding death triggered a reappraisal for some clients who grappled, searched, questioned, and

G. Harvey, *Fundamentalist Religious Childhoods and Adult Mental Health and Wellbeing*, https://doi.org/10.1007/978-3-032-20140-9_8

doubted. Yet, belief in an afterlife, continuing bonds, and religious rituals such as funerals brought comfort and hope. Some of the clients that the participant counsellors had worked with found that spirituality provided a meaning-making system through beliefs and the religion's holy scriptures. One of the main themes in the findings was that spirituality was a coping resource, the sub-themes being the clients' relationship with the divine, including 'leaning on God as a source of strength and comfort' (Johnson & Armour, 2016, p. 277), finding support in their religious community, and religious coping behaviours such as prayer and reading the scriptures. This strengthens Rentzenbrink's (2017, p. 101) perspective that 'religions … are coping strategies. They're people trying to find explanations, rationalise their existences, deal with pain, and work out how to live'.

The conceptualisation of a religious upbringing as beneficial to adult health is unsurprising, given that children are likely to be subjected to the teachings, attend their parents' religious community, and be involved in the common practices. The assertion that the psychological health of religious fundamentalists is positive (Ineichen, 2019, p. 661) backs this up, demonstrating that collective self-esteem and in-group identification (Saroglou, 2011, p. 1322) can be beneficial to wellbeing. This supports the general findings on the positive effects of religion on health and correlates with Heimlich's (2011, p. 23) view that a 'religious upbringing can be a wonderful experience for a child' as it offers connection. It is important to acknowledge that, despite the common view of religious fundamentalism as 'close-minded' (Carlucci et al., 2015, pp. 23–33), it can benefit wellbeing if a child has close bonds with loving parents, enabling the development of healthy brain tissue and creating well-regulated nervous systems (Gerhardt, 2015). A responsive caregiver can also help the child develop healthy re-regulatory responses to stressors, facilitating the growth of resilience (Waite & Ryan, 2020). One early childhood longitudinal study of over 15,000 participants found that parental religious attendance related to fewer behavioural problems with their offspring, with better social interaction and cognitive functioning (Bartkowski et al., 2008), although outcomes on young people's physical health are varied (Oman and Thoreson, 2006).

Yet, what about those who were powerfully controlled by restrictive religion, whose family lives were enmeshed within a religious community where a parent's priority attachment was God, or who suffered religious maltreatment because of a fearful, authoritarian child-rearing style?

The Effects of Developmental Religious Abuse

The lack of choice highlights the injustice of developmental religious abuse. Pasquale (2015) recognises that the brain is very pliable in the early years because its structure is only partially developed, as is the emotional and psychological state. This correlates with Furnari's (2005) assertion that early traumas can negatively affect brain development.

Winell's (n.d.) chart, shown in Fig. 8.1, sets out the restricted conditions for children who grew up in Christianity with hierarchical and patriarchal religious systems embedded in fundamentalism. The figure names this as a closed religious environment where family and church have great authority. Harmful practices are carried out such as unrealistic high standards, isolation, and punishment, together with teachings about fantastical and idealistic doctrines, for example, end times, evil, and damnation, while critical thinking is discouraged, other viewpoints are blocked, and information on science, sex, politics, history, culture, and psychology are withheld, with emotional, intellectual, sexual, and social developmental delays resulting. There are similarities between this and the abuse of children wheel (Domestic Abuse Intervention Programs, 2025) (for example, see Chapter 7). In addition, Cook et al's. (2005) diagram clearly demonstrates the extent to which developmental trauma can impair the domains of a person's biology, affect regulation, alterations to consciousness such as dissociation, attaching to others, control of behaviour, cognition and the self-concept.

The stance that children will be resilient to these enforced conditions is weak against arguments that religious maltreatment by 'frightened and frightening parents' (Golding, 2020, p. 371) can cause developmental trauma. This is not formally diagnosed, but can lead to up to seven areas of impairment. In agreement, Winell (1993, 2016) alleges that religious trauma syndrome (RTS) is now an accepted variant of

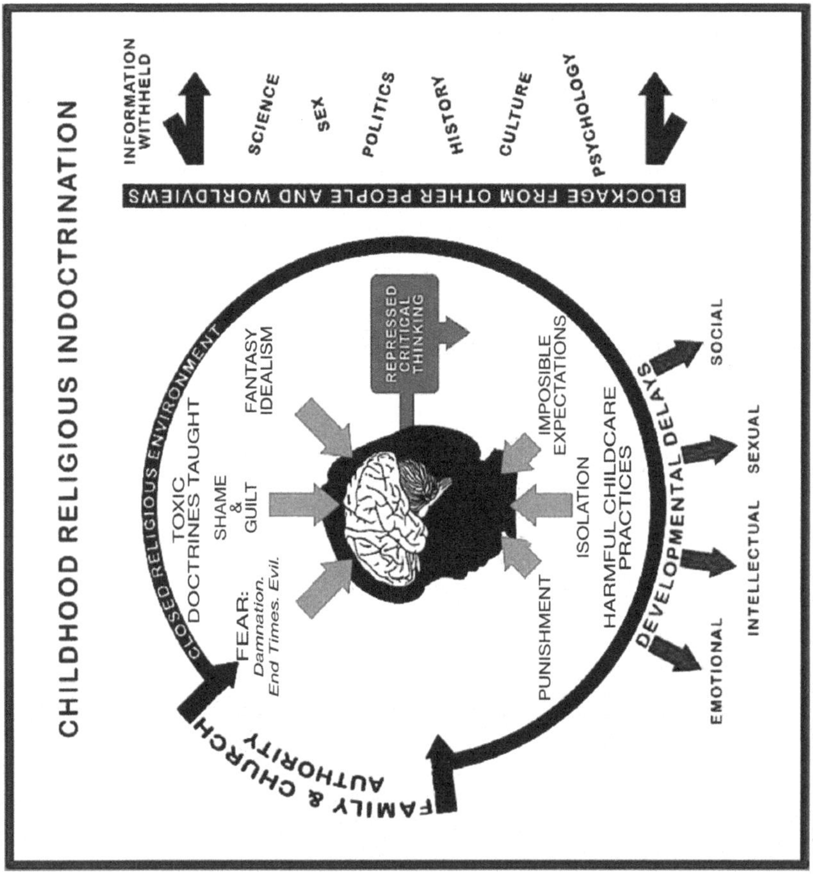

Fig. 8.1 Childhood religious indoctrination (Winell, n.d.)

post-traumatic stress disorder (PTSD), following the combination of strict religious indoctrination on cognitive development in childhood, combined with the trauma of leaving a religious environment in later life. This is thought-provoking, given that writers commonly understand religious and spiritual abuse as occurring in a group or organisational setting (Oakley & Kinmond, 2013; Swindle, 2017), rather than in the home environment or in parallel. However, there is general agreement that, regardless of where it occurs, spiritual abuse can have 'physical, sexual and/or emotional abuse' elements (Cashwell & Swindle, 2018, p. 183). Wherever it happens, it is vital to recognise that while it does not leave any marks on the body (unless it is accompanied by physical and/or sexual abuse), it should not be underestimated since 'spiritual, emotional/psychological, physical, and relational harm' (Roudkovski, 2024, p. 114) occurs in some cases. Francesca Alexandra exemplifies this, as it has greatly affected her health.

> *Looking back, I was plagued by fear, terror, anxiety, bouts of depression, anger (sometimes rage), no voice, difficulty thinking for myself, difficulty knowing my needs/wants, denying myself, poor autonomy, no/little sense of self, difficulty regulating my emotions: on the whole, I shut off emotions apart from happiness.*

She is convinced that because she lived in constant hyper-arousal,[1] there is a legacy of ill health, as her immune system was detrimentally impacted. She struggles with several physical health conditions, including trigeminal neuralgia, cardiac, and rheumatoid issues. Her mental health challenges have included anxiety from a young age, post-natal depression, which she believes could have been diagnosed as psychosis (she was afraid to go to the GP, who could have been the anti-Christ), and undiagnosed complex post-traumatic symptoms, including having nightmares of telephoning 999 but no one answering. Ongoing effects include having difficulty believing she is in pain because she was taught not to trust her feelings, and becoming stressed when questioned by a doctor or her supervisor, who are authority figures for her.

[1] Hyper-arousal is 'a state of heightened physiological and psychological stress, which may result in anxiety, fatigue, and reduced tolerance to pain' (Collins English Dictionary, 2021).

Bearing in mind Heimlich's (2011) criticism of child-rearing practices within fundamentalist Christianity, the North American Committee for Religious Trauma Research (NACRTR) (2020) definition of religious trauma is robustly strong, especially as it is not limited to one form of religious expression and includes the longer-term effects of physical, mental, social, emotional, and spiritual developmental trauma (Duffell & Basset, 2016). Herman (2015) maintains that recurrent childhood trauma deforms the young personality, while Duffell and Basset (2016, p. 26) agree that trauma during the developmental years is stressful and impoverishes 'relational brain tissue', and this is proven in the increased neuroscientific understanding of the brain through advanced imaging in recent years. These texts relay the injurious effects of toxic stress on the body's release of damaging hormones in the growing-up years (Blitz et al., 2016; Shonkoff & Garner, 2012) because of the constant activation of the autonomic nervous system that disrupts many of the bodily systems during sensitive developmental periods (Waite & Ryan, 2020, p. 15). This parallels the original Adverse Childhood Experiences (ACEs) (Felitti et al., 1998) which established a link between health and the ACEs of verbal, physical, and sexual abuse; physical and emotional neglect; the witnessing of domestic violence; substance abuse in the home; separated or divorced parents; and/or a family member in prison or mentally ill or suicidal. The outcomes of this self-reported questionnaire-based research of 1,700 respondents discovered that a greater number of ACEs correlated with a higher level of medical care needed in adulthood. While this study can be critiqued for being a community sample carried out by epistemologists rather than clinical researchers, the omission of many contributory factors to developmental trauma such as relational abuse, poverty, racism, and discrimination such as homophobia, and the failure to investigate factors such as the duration of the adverse experience or the child's age when the event/s occurred, this was groundbreaking seminal work. Newer ACE studies (Bellis et al., 2014; Felitti et al., 2019; Sachs-Ericsson et al., 2017) have made similar links between ACEs and emotional pain becoming physical, as being among the leading causes of death. Sanderson (2020) details the detrimental impact of ACEs as multidirectional, disrupting brain development, the immune and hormonal systems, and the epigenetic code, and impairing social, emotional, and cognitive functioning, while triggering risky health behaviours and causing illness, disability, social problems, and early death caused by sickness and suicide completion. Although developmental religious trauma is not addressed in the original ACEs study (Felitti et al., 1998), it could be present, given the commonly identified factors of closed-minded rigidity, legalistic dogma, authoritarian disciplining, prejudice towards others, separation from the secular world, and the creation of compliance through fear (Hansen, 1998). Trauma, in all its diversity, has the potential to impact every area of a survivor's life. This will be discussed in the next part of this chapter.

The Impact of Trauma on the Six Areas of Functioning

The Waverley Integrative Framework (WIF) is a Christian model that shows the impact on six areas of functioning: physical, emotional, rational, volitional, relational, and spiritual (Kallmier, 2011).

Physical Area of Functioning

Rothschild (2000, p. 5) says that 'trauma is a psychophysical experience, even when the traumatic event causes no direct bodily harm' and there are no visible physical scars. Yet, bodies and brains are geared towards survival, with the amygdala, located in the limbic brain, primed to react to any perceived danger. Van Der Kolk (2014) states that the nervous system behaves differently in traumatic events as the primal area of the brain, situated in the brain stem, is triggered into a fight, flight, freeze, flop, or fawn reaction in a bid to deal with the chaotic consequences. Consequently, a person may be lethargic, listless, and fatigued because so much energy has been invested in survival. Some victims develop psychosomatic conditions such as myalgic encephalomyelitis/chronic fatigue syndrome (ME/CFS) and/or fibromyalgia, especially if there is a culmination of traumatic incidents. McConnaughey (2022, *p. 30) astutely includes*[2] *epigenetics and highlights the research that is being carried out on the effects of trauma on 'gene expression' and how epigenetic changes may help to explain many physical and mental long-term effects.*

While the findings of this study do not focus on themes, cause and effect, or correlations, but commonalities and differences in co-researchers' stories, Table 8.1 shows that while Hannah and Rupert simply described their physical health as good, the remaining participants had various physical health challenges. This is notable as it is consistent with the ACEs research findings. All of the co-researchers, apart from Hannah and Rupert, had experienced Adverse Religious Experiences (AREs).

Table 8.1 Co-researchers' physical health

Pseudonym	Physical health
Holly	Generally well, but has some physical illness, e.g. gall bladder problems
Francesca Alexandra	Described herself as having been 'plagued with different kinds of medical stuff'. Cardiac problems, trigeminal neuralgia, and rheumatoid-type issues. Held the belief that there is a long-term effect on the immune system
Hannah	Good
Eva	Thyroid packed up plus visible goitre ('thankfully benign') when under great family strain, and a trapped nerve in her arm just before leaving the JWs
Anna	Talked about the physical impact of emotional suppression and holding in all the tension for many years
Rupert	Good
Maya	Used to have migraines, nausea, and was sometimes sick when triggered. It was rage that would trigger the migraines. 'It's almost like my body wanted to expel all the trauma and violence, and I was just walking around dazed and floored by all of it'

[2] Epigenetics refers to the way your behaviours and environment can cause changes that affect the way your genes work.

The Emotional, Rational, and Volitional Areas of Functioning

Van Der Kolk's (2014) perspective that trauma affects our physicality, including our immune systems, as well as our emotions and psychological health, correlates with the results of this study. *Effects on these areas of functioning were discovered in the lives of the majority of participants.* Holly faced mental health problems in her teenage years when she was very depressed and emotionally shut down for a long time because she was unable to share her feelings. She took an overdose when she was thirteen years old and has had several breakdowns in adulthood.

The area in the brain responsible for managing emotional response is the amygdala. It directs how to react to situations, commonly without conscious realisation, and is the storehouse of all experience, good, and bad. It remembers how an experience felt and not the factual details. When a person is experiencing an event that is perceived as traumatic, stress hormones are released that govern the fight, flight, or freeze reactions. These stop the hippocampus (the part of the brain thought to be the centre of emotion, memory, and the autonomic nervous system) from working and distort or even delete the facts of the event, the times, and the order of how things happened. An inaccurate record of the event is created which can cause the hippocampus to think that the event is continuing, despite the situation being calm and safe again (Rothschild, 2010) and understanding how these two areas of the brain work together is important, as it is when the hippocampus stops working properly and the felt aspect of an event takes precedence that problems can occur and emotional distress increases. *The level and type of emotional distress experienced will vary from person to person.* A literature review related to chronic stress, including traumatic events, found 'that individuals exposed to trauma frequently experience co-morbid disorders, such as anxiety, depression and PTSD' (D'Andrea et al., 2011, p. 387). When suffering emotional distress, people may not think clearly or make rational decisions because many trauma survivors have an inaccurate or damaged connection to their emotions (McConnaughey, 2022).

While the physical and emotional effects of trauma might be evident, changes in a person's thinking may not be obvious. Van Der Kolk (2014,

p. 21) states that 'it changes not only how we think and what we think about, but also our very capacity to think'. Physiological changes occur alongside, with 'the alarm system being recalibrated, stress hormones increasing, and changes in the system that filters relevant information from irrelevant' (Van der Kolk, 2014, p. 2). Research by Miller et al. (2017) into hippocampus-dependent processes identified an important link between trauma and spatial processing, with a decreased ability to understand and interact with spatial relationships between objects and oneself, potentially eroding confidence and independence.

The effect on the volitional area of functioning involves choices, behaviours, and decision-making. Children growing up in a strict religion will have behavioural expectations prescribed to them at the time when they are also trying to make sense of the world and going through puberty, while their true selves are being flattened. Teaching on sin, hell, and damnation may stop protective decisions from being made or the adoption of healthy coping strategies for fear of punishment. Table 8.2 sets out the co-researchers' mental health at the time of the research interviews. Some, including Holly, Francesca Alexandra, and Maya, described symptoms suggestive of complex post-traumatic stress disorder (C-PTSD), although none had an official diagnosis. Some co-researchers struggled with their mental health from a young age: Maya from about five or six years old, and Holly, who overdosed in her early teens. Francesca Alexandra always had anxiety, but suffered severe paranoia and psychotic-like symptoms after her first child was born. Anna was 'nervous' as a young person and said that terror, fear, nervousness, and anxiety could still 'bubble up' for her. Despite Rupert's positive attitude towards his childhood, he became fearful and anxious when he reached the same age as his mother had been when she had a mental breakdown.

Table 8.2 Co-researchers' mental health

Pseudonym	Mental health
Holly	Depression—very depressed at age thirteen/fourteen years. Overdosed age of thirteen years Various breakdowns (lost language and thought). The biggest breakdown was due to her affair and marital breakdown
Francesca Alexandra	Always had anxiety—became hypervigilant in childhood (aware that she anxiously checked whether her therapist was okay in adulthood) Late twenties, six months after birth of first child, suffered depression with psychotic-like symptoms Complex post-traumatic symptoms (undiagnosed) Severe fear/paranoia (was unable to go to GP as feared she feared the latter was 'the anti-Christ') Pathological caretaking from a young age Used to have severe nightmares, sleepwalking, and great anger
Hannah	Good
Olivia (withdrew at analysis stage)	Not applicable
Eva	'Nearly had a breakdown' at a time of great emotional strain Became depressed and felt hopeless when she thought she was in the JW organisation for the rest of her life
Anna	Nervous as a young person Terror, fear, nervousness, and anxiety can still 'bubble up' Fear of punishment is now rare but can still occur Near-death experience—moments of feeling sick and shame washing over me led to depression and darkness for years. She knew she could not complete suicide because she would go to hell (huge fear) Having to stop bad thoughts because God knows what they are = heavy language and judgement

(continued)

Table 8.2 (continued)

Pseudonym	Mental health
Rupert	Has mostly been positive in life, but had a time of fear and anxiety when he reached the same age as when a parent had a breakdown
Maya	Had very poor mental health as a child, teenager, and adult Depression from a young age (five or six) up until her early twenties Anxiety from five or six years old Undiagnosed PTSD Felt like she was going to explode, needed to get out of those situations, or she would get very aggressive

The Relational Area of Functioning

> Abuse happens at the hands of people we trust, who are supposed to protect us, who represent a God who is all present, all knowing, all powerful. (McBride, 2025, loc. 163)

Anderson (2023, pp. 11–12) shares her story of 'accepting Jesus into her heart on the first day of kindergarten' but later being groomed by the youth pastor, whom she should have been able to trust. This betrayal trauma can severely impact the relational area of functioning.

The teachings based on the holy texts about the expectations of men and women within marriage can profoundly affect relationships more generally. Holly explained her parents' relationship.

> *And when I was thinking about Mum's marriage, which was primarily based on church, they didn't do any fun, they never had a date, they must have had sex because they had a number of children quite quickly, and they prayed every morning, so they read the Bible and you know the alarm went off at six every morning and they prayed and read the Bible every morning, and I think that was part of their connection.*

Francesca Alexandra recognised the damaging impact on familial relationships. She was angry with her mother for a long time and still protected herself as an adult.

> *She is narcissistic with a fragile sense of self, which has triggered her holding on to the rigidity of fundamentalism, which she still does.*

She also acknowledged the impact on her brothers, who struggled with prison, violence, and alcoholism. She was estranged from her younger brother for some years, but he got in touch again during the COVID-19 pandemic because he was convinced that the devil was after him.

Holly revealed that she and her first husband complied with the strict rules about not having sex before marriage, but then their relationship was not consummated for a considerable time. She believes that the detrimental impact continued, and the relationship broke down after her affair was discovered. She felt very judged by Christian friends who disowned her, and she experienced further isolation as a divorced Christian. She talked about her work with clients who had experienced sexual difficulties as a result of their fundamentalist childhoods.

> *I suppose when you're working with couples, and they've had quirky sex, or they haven't had sex, some of them … it's the normality of difficult relationships. They weren't allowed to be together, and then they were allowed to be together, so they've been together seven years, and they've clearly not been having sex or not having penetrative sex … this then affects the rest of their relationship.*

Holly talked about her work as a sex therapist with couples and the impact of fundamentalist religion on relational intimacy.

> *… so by the time she got married in her 30s, she had no sexual feelings. He had a lot of sexual feelings and had watched lots of porn.*

The recognition of the suppression of sexual instincts outside of marriage is apparent in stories. Rupert shared a couple of client situations where the effects of dogmatic beliefs and teaching led to conflict for someone who identified as gay, and another who had 'committed adultery'[3] by having an affair, and who was confused about forgiveness.

The Spiritual/Religious Area of Functioning

> For someone like me, to be wounded spiritually is the worst kind of injury to experience. While other abuses, injuries, and adverse life experiences may take place, the spiritual injury can most poisonously sting at the core of our existence (Marich, 2024, p. 5)

The spiritual area of functioning lies at a person's core and has been called the sacred space of the soul (Pasquale, 2015). *When a person's assumptive world*[4] *is rocked by traumatic abuse, their sense of security, purpose, and meaning can be shaken.* This is conceptualised in the WIF as security, significance, and self-worth (Kallmier, 2011), and their relationship with God (Allah) might also be detrimentally impacted. McChesney (2025, p. xii) refers to 'the notion of soul trauma and its related construct of spiritual injury' and discusses 'the relatively recent construct of "moral injury" because it is widely linked with spirituality'. Anna had a near-death experience, which was 'a time of real crisis', leading to existential grappling. McConnaughey (2022) acknowledges the harmful impact of trauma on trust in the divine (God or Allah) and religious practices such as prayer, concluding that these issues are not spiritual failures but reactions to unresolved traumatic religious events.

---

[3] The committing of adultery is against one of the ten commandments of the Christian Bible (Exodus 20:14).

[4] 'those core beliefs and assumptions that anchor and guide people through life and its many challenges' (Kauffman, 2002, cited in McBeath & Greenlees).

The Effects of Developmental Religious Trauma in Later Life

Very few research studies exist which have examined the impact of a religious fundamentalist childhood on wellbeing in later life, one rare exception being Mytton's (2013) research with those brought up within the Exclusive Brethren religious group, which utilised a 10-point rating scale (10 being the highest level of trauma and 1 no trauma) and found that not everyone was traumatised, although 43 per cent scored 7 or higher. The outcomes also show significant cognitive impact, including 82 per cent of participants stating that they had been brought up with suppressed independent thinking, and 85 per cent believing that they had to think, behave, and feel as they were told. Likewise, the measures used demonstrate that there were considerably higher levels of emotional suffering and interpersonal challenges among participants than in the general population. Mytton's (2013) research found that twenty-seven per cent of the over 250 former member participants had experienced child abuse; symptoms of emotional strain were notably higher than the rest of the population, with many having interpersonal difficulties and showing signs of having been traumatised. Godina's (2014) qualitative research, concerned with reported parenting styles within the Seventh-day Adventist faith, was designed to enable the UK social work profession to increase sensitivity to the spiritual needs of clients. While the findings are informatively thought-provoking, they do not explicitly inform the counselling profession or related caring occupations, although, unlike much of the research on religion and health, people of colour participated. During the literature search for this study, no research was discovered that specifically investigated counsellors' experiences of the influence of a fundamentalist religious upbringing on mental health and wellbeing in adulthood. Many of the papers that exist originate in the USA, with Christianity being the main focus. US Christianity differs from its UK counterpart, and consequently, there is limited applicability.

In the research interviews, Holly voiced some of what made her vulnerable and described herself as malleable.

> *I was a hurt child; it's easy to become a Christian.*

She explained that the emphasis on humans as sinners, rather than unconditional love, facilitated fear and shame. She was convinced that religion can become an addiction, as from an early age she felt compelled to attend church every Sunday and be constantly busy. Holly is certain that the strict religious environment suppressed her natural development and maturation, being compelled to:

> *... leave my brain at the church door, you know, depression not being allowed or questions being allowed ... belief in God wasn't really questioned, the Bible was read literally.*

Holly believes that this impacted many of her life choices. She was a church leader and was in Christian work for most of her life. Her choice of churches in adulthood was also affected.

> *At about 20 years old, I attended a fundamentalist, evangelical, charismatic church who were right about everything, no questioning of faith, no sex before marriage, no real friends outside of the church, with yoga and similar activities all being considered bad. At another stage, when I was in my early 30s, in a fundamentalist church, I recalled thinking that all the people who were not Christians were dangerous to be friends with.*

Co-researcher Eva recalled the impact of being in a clothes shop as a teenager with no idea of what she liked. Francesca Alexandra also spoke about feeling similarly naïve, saying that she had:

> *... poor autonomy, poor skills in autonomous thinking, feeling like an alien in the world with no idea how the world worked or how to defend myself within it, how to relate to it – to people in it. I was denied non-Christian music, radio and tv and have a gap of a decade ... An alien in a foreign land – not belonging, baffling, bewildering, learnt to lie, to wriggle my way out, to be smiley and ever so nice ... we didn't develop at the right time in terms of criticality: there were debating societies at school, and we weren't allowed in them because it would have created disobedience.*

Anna constantly felt guilty as a child and needed to suppress bad thoughts, which was like living in a 'glass box' (Miller, 1987, p. 21). She found God confusing, loving, and comforting but also punishing and wrathful, so the divine being a secure base for her was impossible.

The Effects of Parentification

Family system theorists have long been interested in the concept of parentification, where role-reversal happens prematurely, and children have to take on caregiving roles to enable the family to continue to function and meet parents' needs (Boszormenyi-Nagy & Spark, 1973). Minuchin et al. (1967) describe this as taking on adult responsibilities beyond the child's capacity. One type of parentification involves meeting the emotional needs of a family member in being a confidant, peacemaker, or mediator (Jurkovic et al. 1991, cited in Chase, 1999), while the other is instrumental, involving practical tasks such as washing, ironing, cooking, or helping the parent to shower. The emotional strain leads to greater distress for the young person, with instrumental (helping with practical tasks) (McMahon & Luthar, 2007) less so. Yet both can severely affect a child's psychosocial wellbeing (Castro et al., 2004).

Holly's mother was ill for most of Holly's formative years, necessitating long periods of hospital stays. Consequently, the co-researcher and brother became carers, as their father was usually absent during the daytime. It is possible that the teaching about 'honouring parents'[5] influenced the role-reversed parent–child relationship, as four out of the seven participants (Holly, Francesca Alexandra, Eva, and Rupert) had a family member with serious physical or mental health challenges in their growing-up years.

There are still many unanswered questions about the impact of this on co-researchers' future health, especially for Francesca Alexandra, who described herself as a 'pathological caregiver' from a young age.

[5] Passages about children honouring parents appear in various places in the Bible, with the most recognised one being Matthew 15:4: 'Honour your father and mother' where the scripture talks about respecting and obeying parents.

> *I became the family caretaker, particularly for my Mum's mental health, so she'd spend hours crying, I'd be the one who would stroke her head, I'd be cooking dinner, I'd be cleaning the house … I was seeing home as a safe place when actually it was a prison.*

Research has shown that '75% of young caregivers develop mental health problems including depression, anxiety and low self-esteem' (Frank et al., 1999, cited in Shifren & Kachorek, 2003, p. 339). Moreover, they are likely to engage in risky behaviours such as addiction to substances and be sexually active at a young age, which can add to their health challenges (Stein & Radel, 2004).

The Effects of the Loss of Religious Family and Community

As outlined in Chapter 3, shunning and ostracism have been identified as 'one of the worst things that can happen to a human' (Zieman, 2018 cited in Harvey, 2020, p. 7) which is not surprising, given that 'four fundamental human needs: the need for belonging, self-esteem, control and meaningful existence' (Gutgsell, 2017) are affected. Most of the literature on this topic is biased towards those who leave minority religions, such as the JWs (Frisk, 2018), religious cults, or sects like the Amish in the USA, rather than being applied additionally to churches, mosques, or synagogues. The stigmatisation of those who leave religious groups can increase if they become atheists, especially if they live in predominantly fundamentalist Christian areas such as the Bible Belt in America. This is also largely ignored apart from texts about cults, which is an important oversight, bearing in mind that one US comparison study, which looked at the adult health of 'atheists, agnostics, religious non-affiliated theists, and theistic members of organised religious traditions' found that atheists had the best health outcomes (Baker et al., 2018, p. 44). Psychological turmoil and emotional pain can ensue (Berger, 2015; Fazzino, 2014; Fenelon & Danielsen, 2016; lannaccone, 1994) as Eva explained.

> *I'm very strong, resilient and it's all okay and I've got freedom, I'm building a new life, and I can say all of that, but the reality is, it's heartbreaking because I've lost everything and at my age of nearly 40 how do you rebuild your life ... I've definitely had my moments this year, I've felt completely alone, and those feelings become overwhelming, and you think, do I actually feel a bit suicidal?*

This highlights how important it is that those who have exited fundamentalist religious groups build a non-religious support network (Nica, 2019; Zieman, 2018). There is a parallel between Eva, who was brought up in the JW religion, the only participant to have been shunned after she left, and this subject being largely absent from the literature, apart from papers about cults and minority religions, usually the JWs (Frisk, 2018).

One study 'explored individuals' experiences of religious ostracism' (Gutgsell, 2017, p. 8) using case studies. Unsurprisingly:

> ... participants experienced a decrease in their psychological well-being and some developed psychological disorders during or following the disfellowshipping. Several participants spoke about a lifelong lasting effect. (Gutgsell, 2017, p. 70)

The enormity of this might be comprehended through the 'dimensions of existence' hierarchy (Van Durzen, 2009, p. 84), as ostracism pervades all four dimensions of existence—the physical, social, personal, and spiritual realms. Secondly, polyvagal theory (Porges, 2017) posits that a person who is exiting a cult and being shunned is likely to oscillate between the fight/flight zone (hyper-arousal) and freeze (hypo-arousal). Operating in this way is a primal short-term survival mechanism; however, when this becomes a more permanent 'modus operandi', it is likely to be detrimental to health and wellbeing. The cruel irony is that while being in what is depicted as the green zone, the regulated, safe place, facilitates social engagement, a lack of it (a common consequence of ostracism) can render it impossible to be in the green zone at all. Vastly different emotions are experienced when functioning in the red zone (Spring, 2019) of dorsal vagal hypo-arousal of the ultimate survival of the freeze reaction to the sympathetic fight, flight, in what is depicted as the yellow zone on the polyvagal chart.

Shunning has been described as 'a dark, winding and very lonely path' (Mohammed, 2019, p. 24) because:

> … even in the context of suffering – poverty, violence, human rights violations – not belonging in our families is still one of the most dangerous hurts. That's because it has the power to break our heart, our spirit, and our sense of self-worth. (Brown, 2017, p. 14)

Despite this, Maya emphasised the importance of recognising that it was not all bad.

> *Very little good with the bad outweighing the amount of good … and I think that's also very important to remember, that there were some good things.*

This is why it is important to look at 'both sides of the coin' throughout this publication, and in Chapter 9, the focus will be on healing and recovery.

References

Anderson, L. E. (2023). *When religion hurts you. Healing from religious trauma and the impact of high-control religion*. Brazos Press.

Baker, J. O., Stroope, S., & Walker, M. H. (2018). Secularity, religiosity, and health: Physical and mental health differences between atheists, agnostics, and nonaffiliated theists compared to religiously affiliated individuals. *Social Science Research, 75*, 44–57. https://doi.org/10.1016/j.ssresearch.2018.07.003

Bartkowski, J. P., Xu, X., & Levin, M. L. (2008). Religion and child development: Evidence from the Early Childhood Longitudinal Study. *Social Science Research, 37*, 18–36. https://doi.org/10.1016/j.ssresearch.2007.02.001

Bellis, M. A., Hughes, K., Leckenby, N., Hardcastle, K. A., Perkins, C., & Lowey, H. (2014). Measuring mortality and the burden of adult disease associated with adverse childhood experiences in England: A national survey.

Journal of Public Health, 37(3), 445–454. https://doi.org/10.1093/pubmed/fdu065

Berger, R. (2015). Challenges and coping strategies in leavening an ultra-Orthodox community. *Qualitative Social Work, 14*(5), 670–686. https://doi.org/10.1177/1473325014565147

Blitz, L. V., Anderson, E. M., & Saastamoinen, M. (2016). Assessing perceptions of culture and trauma in an elementary school: Informing a model for culturally responsive trauma-informed schools. *The Urban Review, 48*(4), 520–542. https://doi.org/10.1007/s11256-016-0366-9

Boszormenyi-Nagy, L., & Spark, G. (1973). *Invisible loyalties: Reciprocity in intergenerational family therapy.* Harper & Row.

Brown, B. (2017). *Braving the wilderness. The quest for true belonging and the courage to stand alone.* Vermilion.

Carlucci, L., Tommasi, M., Balsamo, M., Furnham, A., & Saggino, A. (2015). Religious fundamentalism and psychological well-being: An Italian study. *Journal of Psychology and Theology, 43*(1), 23–33. https://doi.org/10.1177/009164711504300103

Cashwell, C. S., & Swindle, P. J. (2018). When religion hurts: Supervising cases of religious abuse. *The Clinical Supervisor, 37*(1), 182–203. https://doi.org/10.1080/07325223.2018.1443305

Castro, D., Jones, R., & Mirsalimi, H. (2004). Parentification and the imposter phenomenon: An empirical investigation. *American Journal of Family Therapy, 32*(1), 205–216.

CDC Genomics and Your Health. Epigenetics, Health, and Disease. https://www.cdc.gov/genomics-and-health/epigenetics/index.html

Chase, N. (1999). *Burdened children: Theory, research and treatment.* SAGE. https://www.google.co.uk/books/edition/Burdened_Children/4qjOCQAAQBAJ?hl=en&gbpv=1.

Collins English Dictionary. (2019). https://www.collinsdictionary.com/dictionary/english/abrahamic

Cook, A., Spinazzola, J., & Ford, J. (2005). Complex trauma in children and adolescents. *Psychiatric Annals, 35*, 395–398.

D'Andrea, W., Sharma, R., Zelecheski, A. D., & Spinazzola, J. (2011). Physical Health Problems After Single Trauma Explosure: When Stress Takes Root in the Body. *Journal of the American Psychiatric Nurses Association, 17*(6), 378–392.

Domestic Abuse Intervention Programs. (2025). https://www.TheDuluthModel.org

Duffell, N., & Basset, T. (2016). *Trauma, abandonment and privilege*. Routledge.

Fazzino, L. L. (2014). Leaving the church behind: Applying a deconversion perspective to evangelical exit narratives. *Journal of Contemporary Religion, 29*(2), 249–266. https://doi.org/10.1080/13537903.2014.903664

Felitti, V., Anda, R., Nordenberg, D., Williamson, D., Spitz, A., Edwards, V., Koss, M., & Marks, J. (1998). Relationship of childhood abuse and household dysfunction to many of the leading causes of death in adults. *American Journal of Preventative Medicine, 14*(4), 245–258. https://doi.org/10.1016/S0749-3797(98)00017-8

Felitti, V. J., Anda, R. F., Nordenberg, D., Williamson, D. F., Spitz, A. M., Edwards, V., Koss M. P., & Marks, J. S. (2019). Reprint of: Relationship of childhood abuse and household dysfunction to many of the leading causes of death in adults: The adverse childhood experiences (ACE) study. *American Journal of Preventive Medicine, 56*(6), 774–786. https://doi.org/10.1016/j.amepre.2019.04.001

Fenelon, A., & Danielsen, S. (2016). Leaving my religion: Understanding the relationship between religious disaffiliation, health, and well-being. *Social Science Research, 57*, 49–62. https://doi.org/10.1016/j.ssresearch.2016.01.007

Frisk, L. (2018). Diana Baumrind's parenting styles: Examples of the Osho movement and Jehovah's Witnesses. In L. Frisk, S. Nilsson, & P. Akerback (Eds.), *Children in minority religions. Growing up in controversial religious groups* (pp. 149–170). Equinox.

Furnari, L. (2005). Born or raised in closed, high-demand groups: Developmental considerations. *ICSA e-newsletter, 4*(3). https://www.spiritualabuseresources.com/articles/born-or-raised-in-closed-high-demand-groups-developmental-considerations

Gerhardt, S. (2015). *Why love matters. How affection shapes a baby's brain.* Routledge.

Godina, L. (2014). Religion and parenting: Ignored relationship? *Child and Family Social Work, 19*, 381–390. https://doi.org/10.1111/cfs.12054

Golding, K. S. (2020). Understanding and helping children who have experienced maltreatment. *Paediatrics and Child Health, 30*(11), 371–377. https://doi.org/10.1016/j.paed.2020.08.002

Gutgsell, J. (2017). *A loving provision? How former Jehovah's Witnesses experience shunning* (Master's thesis, Vrije Universiteit Brussels, Brussels). https://saysorry.org/wp-content/uploads/2019/09/shunning-and-disfellowshipping-in-jehovahswitnesses-by-j-gutgsell.pdf

Hansen, C. (1998). Long-term effects of religious upbringing. *Mental Health, Religion and Culture, 1*(2), 91–111. 1080/13674679808406502

Harvey, G. (2020). Ostracism. *ICSA Today, 11*(3), 7–9.

Harvey, G. M. (2017). An exploration of counsellors' lived experiences of the impact of client spirituality when bereavement is the presenting issue. [Unpublished Master's thesis] Waverley Abbey College, UK.

Heimlich, J. (2011). *Breaking their will. Shedding light on religious child maltreatment*. Prometheus Books.

Herman, J. (2015). *Trauma and recovery. The aftermath of violence from domestic abuse to political terror*. Basic Books.

Iannaccone, L. R. (1994). Why strict churches are strong. *American Journal of Sociology, 99*(5), 1180–1211. https://doi.org/10.1086/230409

Ineichen, B. (2019). Losing the rapture: Escaping from fundamentalist Christian belief. *Mental Health, Religion & Culture, 22*(7), 661–673. https://doi.org/10.1080/13674676.2018.1557872

Johnson, S. K., & Armour, M. P. (2016). Finding strength, comfort, and purpose in spirituality after homicide. *Psychology of Religion and Spirituality., 8*(4), 277–288.

Kallmier, R. (2011). *Caring and counselling.* CWR.

Marich, J. (2024). *You lied to me about God.* North Atlantic Books.

McBeath, A., & Greenlees, P. (2016). Psychological and therapeutic issues associated with membership of high-demand religious groups. *Psychotherapy Section Review, 58*, 71–76.

McBride, H. L. (2025). *Holy hurt. Understanding spiritual trauma and the process of healing*. Brazos Press.

McChesney, R. W. (2025). *The soul also keeps the score. A trauma-informed companion to the spiritual exercises of St. Ignatius.* Liturgical Press.

McConnaughey, J. (2022). *Trauma in the pews. The impact on faith and spiritual practices.* Berry Powell Press.

McMahon, T., & Luthar, S. (2007). Defining characteristics and potential consequences of caretaking burden among children living in urban poverty. *American Journal of Orthopsychiatry, 77*(2), 267–281. https://doi.org/10.1037/0002-9432.77.2.267

Miller, J. K., McDougall, S., Thomas, S., & Wiener, J. M. (2017). Impairment in active navigation from trauma and post-traumatic stress disorder. *Neurobiology of Learning and Memory, 140*, 114–123.

Minuchin, S., Montalvo, B., Guerney, Jr., Rosman, B., & Schumer, F. (1967). *Families of the slums: An exploration of their structure and treatment.* Basic Books.

Mohammed, Y. (2019). *Unveiled. How Western liberals empower radical Islam.* Free Hearts Free Minds.
Mytton, J. (2013). *Second-generation adult survivors of the Hales Exclusive Brethren: Mental health, childhood sexual abuse and interpersonal problems.* Paper presented at The International Cultic Studies Association Annual Conference, Trieste, Italy.
Nica, A. (2019). Exiters of religious fundamentalism: Reconstruction of social support and relationships related to well-being. *Mental Health, Religion & Culture, 22*(5), 543–556. https://doi.org/10.1080/13674676.2019.1636015
Oakley, L., & Kinmond, K. (2013). *Breaking the silence on spiritual abuse.* Palgrave Macmillan.
Oman, D., & Thoresen, C. E. (2006). Religion, spirituality, and children's physical health. In E. C. Roehlkepartain, P. E. King, L. Wagener, & P. L. Benson (Eds.). *The handbook of spiritual development in childhood and adolescence, 399.* Sage. https://doi.org/10.4135/9781412976657.n28
Pasquale, T. B. (2015). *Sacred wounds. A path to healing from spiritual trauma.* Chalice Press.
Porges, S. W. (2017). *The pocket guide to the polyvagal theory: The transformative power of feeling safe.* Norton.
Ransom, H. J., Monk, R. L., & Heim, D. (2021). Grieving the living: The social death of former Jehovah's Witnesses. *Journal of Religion and Health, 61*, 2458–2480. https://doi.org/10.1007/s10943-020-01156-8
Rentzenbrink, C. (2017). *A manual for heartache. How to feel better.* Picador.
Rothschild, B. (2000). *The body remembers.* Norton.
Rothschild, B. (2010). *8 keys to safe trauma recovery. Take-charge strategies to empower your healing.* Norton.
Roudkovski, K. (2024). *Understanding spiritual abuse. What it is and how to respond.* B&H Academic.
Sachs-Ericsson, N. J., Sheffler, J. L., Stanley, I. H., Piazza, J. R., & Preacher, K. J. (2017). When emotional pain becomes physical: Adverse childhood experiences, pain, and the role of mood and anxiety disorders. *Journal of Clinical Psychology, 73*(10), 1403–1428. https://doi.org/10.1002/jclp.22444
Sanderson, C. (2020, June 26). Adverse childhood experiences. *Nscience.*
Saroglou, V. (2011). Believing, bonding, behaving, and belonging: The big four religious dimensions and cultural variation. *Journal of Cross-Cultural Psychology, 42*(8), 1320–1340. https://doi.org/10.1177/0022022111412267
Shifren, K., & Kachorek, L. (2003). Does early caregiving matter? The effects on young caregivers' adult mental health. *International Journal of*

Behavioral Development, 27(4), 338–346. https://doi.org/10.1080/01650250244000371

Shonkoff, J., & Garner, A. (2012). The committee on psychosocial aspects of child and family health, committee on early childhood adoption and dependent care, and section on developmental and behavioral pediatrics. *Pediatrics, 129*(1), 232–246.

Smith, J. A., Flowers, P., & Larkins, M. (2009). *Interpretative phenomenological analysis, theory, method and research*. Sage.

Spring, C. (2019). *Feelings in different zones*. https://www.carolynspring.com/shop/shame-resource-pack/.

Stein, M., & Radel, M. (2004). Parentification and its impact on adolescent children of parents with AIDS. *Family Process, 38*(2), 193–208. https://doi.org/10.1111/j.1545-5300.1999.00193.x

Swindle, P. J. (2017). *A twisting of the sacred: The lived experience of religious abuse* (PhD thesis, University of North Carolina). https://www.proquest.com/docview/1927630238?%20Theses&fromopenview=true&fromunauthdoc=true&pq-origsite=gscholar&sourcetype=Dissertations%20

Van der Kolk, B. (2014). *The body keeps the score*. Penguin Random House.

Van Durzen, E. (2009). *Psychotherapy and the quest for happiness*. Sage.

Van Eck Duymaer van Twist, A. (2015). *Perfect children: Growing up on the religious fringe*. Oxford University Press. https://doi.org/10.1093/acprof.oso/9780199827787.001.0001

Waite, R., & Ryan, R. A. (2020). *Adverse childhood experiences. What students and health professionals need to know*. Routledge.

Winell, M. (1993). *Leaving the fold. A guide for former fundamentalists and others leaving their religion*. Apocryphile Press.

Winell, M. (n.d.). *Factors in childhood indoctrination in fundamentalist Christianity*. http://journeyfree.org/wp-content/uploads/A-GRAPH-Childhood-Indoctrination-color.jpg

Zieman, B. (2018) *Shunned: A survival guide*. Great Britain: Amazon.

9 Healing and Recovery

In this chapter, the co-researchers' stories of recovery from the effects of religious trauma in their developmental years will be shared. For many, their healing only begins once they have exited the fundamentalist religious group, which is a very complicated process and often the polarised opposite experience to 'the good beginning' (Roudkovski, 2024, p. 62) where people are 'love-bombed' (Singer, 2003, pgs. 114–115). Roudkovski's (2024) metaphor of a spider's web signifies what a frightening and confusing departure this can be. Oakley and Humphreys (2019) use the metaphor of getting out of a maze to illustrate the challenge of a powerless member leaving after having been controlled by powerful leaders.

Transitioning into Society

> More often than not, leaving a cult environment requires an adjustment period, not only to reintegrate into 'normal' society but also, to put the pieces of yourself back together in a way that makes sense to you. (Tobias, 1994, cited in Zieman, 2017, pp. 112–113)

G. Harvey, *Fundamentalist Religious Childhoods and Adult Mental Health and Wellbeing*, https://doi.org/10.1007/978-3-032-20140-9_9

This quotation succinctly summarises the challenges of leaving a fundamentalist religious group physically and psychologically, and transitioning into society, some for the first time, while being shunned. One ex-member described it in this way: 'in the Amish, at least you're someone … in the English-speaking world you're a number' (The Amish: Shunned, 2014, 01:45:47). Therefore, 'ostracism … disrupt(s) our sense of ourselves as members of an interconnected human community' (Bastian & Haslam, 2010, p. 107). Additionally, the introjects (Jenkinson, 2019b, p. 14) of the false self (Winnicott, 1965) or cult pseudo-personality (Lifton, 1989), which enabled survival while in the group, are 'shaken to the core' by being 'out in the world' (Jenkinson, 2019a, p. 23). To aid understanding of a very challenging emotional and psychological experience, Zieman (2018, p. 12) identifies what she calls 'the predictable phases of experience': 'shock/disbelief, hurt/loneliness, fear/desperation, struggle, choice points A & B, re-engagement/re-connection, coming to terms with new reality, embracing life'. These resonate hauntingly with well-known stages and phases of grief models, for example, Kübler-Ross (1969) and Kübler-Ross and Kessler (2005). An alternative model suggests three steps of the process: stage 1—safety, stage 2—remembrance and mourning, and stage 3—reconnecting and meaning (Herman, 2015, cited in Zieman, 2017, pp. 15–16).

While these models are helpful, a key critique is the innate suggestion that the phases are linear and time-limited. Kübler-Ross and Kessler (2005, p. 18) state that 'stages are responses for feelings that can last for minutes or hours as we flip in and out of one and then another', and it is plausible that someone who has exited and/or been shunned may go through these processes due to the losses involved.

From her research with cult survivors, Jenkinson (2019b, p. 24) suggests a four-phase approach to recovery. This is robust since she says that 'it is important to emphasise that the phases may need revisiting and are not necessarily linear' (2019a, p. 26). Adults can be classified in three ways: First Generation Adults (FGAs), Second Generation Adults (SGAs) and Multi-Generation Adults (MGAs) will go through different processes:

The FGA will be regaining their sense of self: the SGA (and MGA) may be finding theirs for the first time.

Despite the upsurge of interest in religious trauma:

> … there remains a significant gap in the understanding of how individuals navigate these experiences, derive meaning, and experience PTG (post-traumatic growth) from them. (Perry, 2024, p. 1)

This highlights the importance of those who have left fundamentalist religious groups in establishing a non-religious support network (Nica, 2019; Zieman, 2018).

However, survivors' narratives regarding recovery are crucial to understanding, so the author firstly shares her healing journey, followed by the co-researchers' stories as revealed during the research interviews.

My Healing Journey

> Maybe the journey isn't so much about becoming anything.
> Maybe it's about unbecoming everything that really isn't you
> so, you can become who you were meant to be in the first place. (Paulo Coelho)[1]

It took many years for me to accept the truth regarding the strict control with which I grew up. In my formative years, I was taught that a good Christian always helps others, and it is not surprising that I became a psychotherapist. It was in the 1990s that I became curious about counselling and psychotherapy because I started to realise the power of being listened to and heard, rather than always being told what to do. Driven by a passion to help grieving people, and finding that I was naturally able to listen to others, I trained to be a bereavement listener and enjoyed getting alongside clients.

[1] Attributed to Paulo Coelho and thought to be something he said rather than wrote.

I did not experience counselling until 2002, as I became severely ill with ME/CFS; there was a substantial amount of emotional and psychological baggage that I needed to deal with. Yet, what I experienced as a client was hope that therapy might be helpful in finding better health. This anchored me during an extremely dark time, which echoes Yalom's (2017, p. 219) description of the 'ultimate test of endurance'. I reap the benefits of the realisations that I gained, in the wellbeing that I now enjoy.

Why was that therapeutic experience so pivotal in my journey back to health? I now realise that the counsellor offered the core conditions[2] (Rogers, 1961), which were non-judgemental and accepting. These were monumental because they were the polarised opposite of judgemental, authoritarian, and critical childhood experiences described below:

> all too many of those who seek the help of counsellors have spent much of their lives surrounded by people who with devastating inappropriateness have appointed themselves experts in the conduct of people's lives. (Mearns & Thorne, 2007, p. 10)

It is almost impossible to find words to describe the healing nature of the core conditions when never been experienced before, and I will be eternally grateful that at the core of the counselling lay the counsellor's desire:

> … to provide a different soil and a different climate in which the the client can recover from past deprivation or maltreatment and begin to flourish as the individual he or she is. (Mearns & Thorne, 2007, p. 14)

What I came to realise was that I had introjected the damaging, negative, demeaning childhood messages, and that those beliefs and behaviours had 'remain(ed) sitting in (my) psychological system like a lump of unchewed and undigested food in (the) gut' (Jenkinson, 2019a, 2019b, p. 14). This aligns with Rogers' (1961) view that if a person constantly receives negative reactions and feedback, their innate need for positive regard and approval remains. In my case, I became 'a good girl',

[2] The 'core conditions' of empathy, congruence, and unconditional positive regard.

which I now understand as the forming of a pseudo-personality (Jenkinson, 2008), creating incongruence between my need for approval and my potential:

> … so great is the need in all of us that its satisfaction can take precedence over the promptings of the actualising tendency and as a consequence, creates gross confusion for the organismic valuing process. (Mearns & Thorne, with McCleod, 2013, p. 10)

As I started to explore these deep issues in therapy, especially around the necessity of shedding the pseudo-personality (Jenkinson, 2008), my health plummeted again, and I became extremely ill and housebound once more. Thankfully, the counsellor agreed to weekly telephone sessions. I was encouraged to recognise and express my feelings for the first time. Yet, the most empowering aspect was that the therapist believed in me, and I started to believe in myself and trust that good things could happen to me as well as to everyone else. This signalled a notable shift, and gradually my health began to improve again, and I was able to resume face-to-face counselling sessions. There can be little doubt that the nurturing therapeutic environment was life-changing.

For me, as for many other survivors of religious abuse, this was not the end of the story, and in the intervening years I have healed further, with the journey continuing to the present day, even though I have needed to estrange myself from members of my extended family. The dynamics around the deaths of both my parents have emphasised the pain of no longer belonging in my family of origin.

There have been many physical health challenges over the years, although I have now been free from the symptoms of ME/CFS for many years. I no longer regard myself as religious, as my much-evolved faith brings less rigidity, dogma, and legalism. For years, I felt a spiritual failure, believing that I could not reach the expected standards of being a good Christian. I found it very helpful to discover McConnaughy's (2022) assertion that victims of religious abuse who often regard themselves as spiritual failures are living with trauma responses.

Recent semi-retirement has brought greater opportunity for solitude and silence, alongside sessions with my spiritual director, who is not legalistic or dogmatic and never judges. This has helped me to deconstruct the fundamentalist religious introjects and practices into a far less certain but evolved faith. *At present, I am training to be a spiritual accompanier to others whose souls have been violated, those affected by betrayal trauma, and those suffering the effects of soul injury every day of their lives.*

Table 9.1 outlines the religious/spiritual status of each co-researcher as disclosed at the time of the research interviews.

Four out of seven participants have continued with some of their evolved but foundational beliefs and practices, although this continuation is not the focus of this research. This is of interest because the literature shows that these beliefs and practices can positively influence

Table 9.1 The co-researchers' religious statuses

Pseudonym	Upbringing	Current faith
Holly	Baptist (works with many Muslim clients)	Christian and attends church regularly but is undergoing a faith shift currently
Francesca Alexandra	Pentecostal Christian	Strong Christian faith and a regular church attender
Hannah	Liberal Judaism	Continues to be a practising Jew, which she sees as cultural rather than just religious
Olivia (withdrew at analysis stage)	Pentecostal Christian	Yes
Eva	Jehovah's Witnesses	Left the JWs as an adult. Interested in exploring spirituality later in her life
Anna	Evangelical Baptist	No longer believes in religion but sees herself as 'spiritual'
Rupert	Evangelical Baptist	Continues to be a committed Christian
Maya	Sunni Muslim	No longer a Muslim. Would like to explore spirituality more in due course, but is not ready to do so yet

resilient wellbeing if continued into adult life (Hand, 2002, cited in Koenig & Larson, 2001). Anna now sees herself as spiritual, with Eva and Maya expressing interest in exploring spirituality later in life. Holly still identifies as a Christian but has undergone faith shifts due to revelations following the death of a relative who was viewed as a pillar of the church. This has challenged her faith, which she described at the start of the project as 'the best it has ever been'. While not all of the participants have continued with their childhood beliefs and practices, all are trained counsellors who require great resilience to work with client distress. What enables them to be durable practitioners is unclear, although factors other than religion can enable this.

Co-researchers' Healing and Recovery

Regarding healing and recovery, Marich (2024, p. 5) writes:

> Even though I've spent twenty years on my recovery journey and am a much better version of myself than the girl who left my parents' house in 2000, I am still healing from the wreckage. I am a casualty of this spiritual warfare and the toxic shame it created in me.

The co-researchers were interviewed at different points in their healing. Eva and Maya were in the early stages, Francesca Alexandra was further on, and as mentioned, Holly has since deconstructed and reconstructed her Christian faith. Anna now sees herself as spiritual and shared that she was in a far freer landscape than before. Each recovery journey is unique. A summary will now be given of each co-researcher's reflective feedback following the completion of their involvement in the project.

Hannah

As we have seen, Hannah grew up in liberal, cultural Judaism, and she radiates robustness, with the beliefs, values, and practices learned in childhood continuing to be integral to life as demonstrated in the weekly

Shabbat ritual, which she views as a time of rest that supports her life and that of her family. She reflected on participating in the project.

> *My primary feeling about been involved as a co-researcher has been how I have taken for granted much of what being as a member of a community, that is grounded in religion, has offered me … This has therefore heightened my awareness of how vital a belonging to a religious group can be, as I can both offer and receive support that is crucial to wellbeing at this time.*

Rupert

This co-researcher continues to be a committed Christian, as he has been from a young age. In his written reflections, he recognised that his religious upbringing had elements of fundamentalism in having a specific sacred text and mandating strict adherence to a belief set and rules, but that the effects were ameliorated by love. His participation enabled him to gain new insights.

> *I was humbled by the interview, helping to make me realise how far I've travelled.*

Maya

Although Maya described her emotional robustness as good, she was just beginning her recovery process and was in twice-weekly therapy. Early in the first interview, she was triggered, and her cognition went offline. The research conversation stopped while she was helped to re-ground herself, so that the interview could continue once she had re-regulated. She shared that one of her clients had grown up in a similar situation to hers, although in an African country, which had enabled Maya to recognise her lack of choice and religious freedom in childhood.

> *I am glad this is over and feel proud that I have completed the most difficult part of the process. This has been at times harrowing, incredibly difficult, painful and triggering, however I have been able to work through a great*

deal of the trauma I suffered however, in therapy I have been able to get free from much of what has troubled me, albeit also quite sad … Telling my story to Gill was a crucial part in my being able to come to a place of peace with my past. I will be eternally grateful for being allowed to be part of this very important work. It has been an important part of my healing and has made me feel as though I am not alone and that there is hope. I have gotten so much more out of this than I could have hoped for … And likewise, it saddens me, but it also gives me strength to know that I am not alone in this.

She also stated that participation had brought up many questions and made her curious, but she was working towards shining more light on her shame. As can be seen from the religious statuses table, Maya no longer identifies as a Muslim but said that she is interested in exploring spirituality in the future.

Francesca Alexandra

This co-researcher continues to have a strong faith and regularly attends her church. She believes that this sustains her, as she shared that she is much stronger and now quite peaceful about her history. Yet, she expressed being slightly surprised at the extent of the emotion she felt during the process, despite extensive therapy and healing.

It has been an immensely positive, enriching and precious process, shared process, shared experiences, shared knowing, hearing and being heard, a shared deep understanding of each other's worlds with striking similarities … It has been deeply moving. It has brought more joy as my gratitude has increased further; I am reminded that God has restored the years the locusts had eaten. I feel whole, I feel alive, and more. My own emotions have been deep and varied throughout this process: sadness, anger, gratitude, positivity. In some ways, the process has shown that I still have wounds, but it also shows that I am living well, extremely well. My remaining words serve me well – they are a reminder, but I am not swamped. They connect me deeply to others (my clients, colleagues, God). I am grateful for them. One positive is that I feel deeply, and I connect deeply as a result. I live well because of my past, not despite it.

She shared that it had taken ten years of God healing her, including the words of a Welsh hymn, eighteen months of therapy with an ex-Brethren counsellor, which she described as 'soothing', and her use of humour. She recalled a reparative childhood event when she took back a book she had stolen from the Pastor's bookshelf and was not shamed. As an adult, she attended a national Christian event when a senior church leader apologised for how God had been misrepresented by the church, which had traumatised so many people.

> *God, in His loving wisdom, stepped into my world using one of my languages, which is music*[3] *(a Welsh hymn). He touched me with a whisper, his small voice, and it was love. Through therapy, God's grace, and the church, I have developed and grown incredibly, and I am no longer just surviving – I am thriving. I used to get by in spite of my past, but that is no longer true. I am now thriving and am stronger because of it (not despite it), and I have insight into many of my clients' woundedness as a result. Our traumas don't need to define us; they don't need to be a legacy of destruction. We can use it, and I think that's my gratitude and that was my training ground … I can now be free to be me … and there's gratitude around that. God's provided people who have been able to attend to some of my wounds relationally.*

Some of Francesca Alexandra's healing has been relational, which matches with Marich's (2024, p. 6) perspective.

Until deep levels of healing can take place, that spiritual wounding colours so many human interactions, especially in our closest relationships. Such wounding can make you feel even more unsafe and insecure as you navigate living in this world. Sometimes I can still get overwhelmed trying to sort it all out. In these moments, I must remember to be gentle with myself. This task can be difficult when you were raised with a God that was anything but gentle, or your head became scrambled with all sorts of mixed messages.

---

[3] The Welsh hymn 'Here is love vast as the ocean'/ 'Dyma gariad fel y moroedd'.

Eva

Eva had left the JWs approximately two years before I met her and was also early on in her recovery process. She spoke about her growth since leaving the organisation and acknowledged she was not the same person because she had learned to protect herself. She had experienced 'periods of intense loneliness' since, but said that she had left physically and mentally, so she could never go back. She commented on the importance of learning to hold boundaries.

> *It's okay to put those boundaries in place; it's okay to own your own story and decide what happens from here on in.*

Being understood by her therapist was a key part of her recovery:

> *The feeling of being understood and being heard is massive to the journey of recovery.*

But also commented on the longevity of the healing process:

> *It's never a quick fix to do things and come to a growing understanding of what we have experienced, but just suddenly having the realisation of how it's impacting you takes a long time.*

Being a co-researcher helped Eva to come to terms with seeing the JWs as a fundamentalist religion, alongside acknowledging the indoctrination she was exposed to and its lifelong effect on her emotions and thinking. She summarised her experience in participating.

> *I've really enjoyed the process. It's been really fascinating to connect over these things with somebody that I've never met before. Yes, it's been a real privilege. It brought out some good emotions in me.*

Anna

Anna is now spiritual rather than religious, her position matching Zinnbauer et al.'s assertion (1997 cited in Wortmann & Park, 2008, p. 703) that people who do not identify as religious may identify as spiritual, and with Mathis-Rimes' (2018, pp. 27–28) view of spirituality as having a bond with God/Universe/Source and being focussed on unconditional love. Yet, she spoke about missing being able to go to God in difficult times (Beck & McDonald, 2004, p. 1010).

There was always somewhere to go, you know, so at my most lonely childhood or adolescent places, then yes, sitting at God's knee I could find at times immensely comforting and that as part of the rule that we looked to God as father and we were the children of God, it was easier to just let my mother or God take control.

She described being in a more healing, peaceful place now and was deeply reflective about engaging with the research process.

I was faced, I believe, with a deeper understanding of the reality that my mental health had/has been massively affected by my fundamentalist religious upbringing, and that it continues to affect me. This research process, my personal reflections, disclosures, writing and our shared hours have deepened the respect I have for myself and heightened my appreciation of how terribly sincerely I believed everything I had been taught. No, there was no choice, but (at the time) I would not have wanted a choice.

While she continued to struggle with decision-making and managing finances, she commented on the importance of the research conversations, which she called 'soul reflection'.

So powerful and the healing nature of such deep sharing was powerfully acknowledged by both of us.

Holly

After the end of our work together, Holly's emotional robustness was destabilised by revelations about a recently deceased relative who had been regarded as an upstanding member of the church. Following this, Holly started to deconstruct and reconstruct her faith.

In her musings, Holly thought that her participation had come at the right time because she was in a place where she could reflect.

> *I've found being part of the research cathartic, costly and freeing ... I recognise I had to reflect on the impact of my involvement in fundamentalism and how this had impacted my relationships both socially and at work as a counsellor ... I think the research project has enabled me the time to reflect on the shame I felt by not taking responsibility for my beliefs. I recognise I still feel sad that I stopped thinking, but I understand I was looking for family, identity, purpose and belonging. I lacked confidence, and I looked to others for validation. I can see the clinging influence of my shame, now. I can see this as a work in progress with an option of growing into my beliefs and sense of self. I am aware that as I talk about and tell my story, there is the option of walking into the healing and wholeness of God's love. Like all of us, there are implications of my earlier decisions, but that gives me the richness of life that I now have.*

Holly stated that as part of their recovery:

> *People need to start thinking for themselves, face their darkness, and question ... But the reality is that my experience was that fundamentalism stops the questions and thus the growth and development that questions and disagreement bring. Survivors can gain psycho-education, do some stabilisation, learn grounding skills (ready for flashbacks), and gain a window of tolerance. Then the process stages of telling the story ... vivid and repetition likely ... then integrate the experiences and re-engage with ourselves and the world ... and hold in mind that seventy per cent of people manage post-traumatic growth.*

Post-Traumatic Growth

In the early years, resilience emanates from security with parents as a result of positive attention, rare separation from the attachment figure in infancy, a close bond with their caregivers, and emotional support from outside their family. As we have seen, a child is secure when the adult is responsively accessible to them, so that the child can explore the world based on the consistent and reassuring presence of the caregiver who will provide relief and security when the child is frightened (Harris, 2002). *Conversely, those who grow up in circumstances of little attunement or attention are likely to have insecure bonds and be less resilient in adulthood.* Hardy people also suffer traumatic events, but generally, they can function healthily despite them.

The findings of this research, together with the literature search, have revealed that religious abuse can impact the whole person, leaving them fragile, vulnerable, and unregulated. There are no statistics available to show how often PTG results from trauma (Vazquez et al., 2022, p. 755), but some research has revealed that the religious variables of engagement in deep rumination (DR), attachment to God, and Christian gratitude can be contributory factors to 'transcendent meaning making' (Vis and Boynton (2008, p. 74) for those of a Christian faith after trauma and in life generally. This PTG can increase the capacity to adapt and cope effectively with other difficult circumstances.

Religious abuse causes spiritual injury yet can also be 'an essential component of coping following trauma, including spiritual-distress (SD) related wounds' (De Vynck et al., 2023, p. 2). One scoping literature review (Perry, 2024) recognise that while storytelling might be a central part of post-traumatic growth, additional challenges are commonly present for survivors because 'disbelief, stigmatisation, isolation, shaming and even overt hostility from the public and their communal religious environment are often experienced' (Doyle, 2009; Ellis et al., 2023; Flynn, 2008; Heyder, 2022; Pargament et al., 2008). This resonates with the results of an interpretative phenomenological analysis (IPA) of four female participants with evangelical Christian personal histories who experienced SD (De Vynck et al., 2023 p. 2), Despite the isolation of such experiences, spirituality also played a role in their post-traumatic growth, as they navigated the choppy waters from the certainty of 'the supposed safety and belonging found on the shore of their EC foundation' into uncertainty and 'a profound sense of existential disorientation' (De Vynck et al., 2023, pp. 5–6). Areas of PTG were later noted within their relationships: genuineness, congruence, life appreciation, and spiritual spaciousness (De Vynck et al., 2023, p. 9). Perry (2024, pp. 3–6) observes that three factors facilitated survivors in their recovery: 'recognition: naming the abuse; relaying: exploring the trauma narrative and redefining: transformation of spirituality'. However, it is important to remember that most of the research on SD has used quantitative methodology and has been carried out with white American Christian participants (De Vynck et al., 2023, p. 1). The majority of the co-researchers' stories contain these components, including the changes to their religious statuses as established in Table 9.1.

Counsellors' experiences around the influence of a fundamentalist religious upbringing and the adult effects are varied. The accounts of harm suffered resonate with some of the texts (Blitz et al., 2016; Duffell & Bassett, 2016, pp. 19–26; Herman, 2015, p. 96; Shonkoff & Garner, 2012) about the damaging effects of the toxic stress of developmental trauma, with many of the bodily systems being disrupted (Waite & Ryan, 2020, p. 15). However, it is clear that it is not just the physicality of the young person that is detrimentally impacted by such experiences in the formative years, but that it affects a person 'physically, somatically, emotionally, neurologically, behaviorally, relationally, and even ethically' (Rogers, 2024, p. 1). Chapter 10 will look at the implications for counsellors, psychotherapists, and other practitioners who work with victims of these abusive occurrences.

References

American Experience/PBS. (2014). *The Amish: Shunned* [Video]. YouTube. https://youtube.com/watch?v=zQ0uVZiHX8g

Bastian, B., & Haslam, N. (2010). Excluded from humanity: The dehumanizing effects of social ostracism. *Journal of Experimental Social Psychology, 46*, 107–113.

Beck, R., & McDonald, A. (2004). Attachment to God: The attachment to God inventory, tests of working model correspondence, and an exploration of faith group differences. *Journal of Psychology and Theology, 32*(2), 92–103. https://doi.org/10.1177/009164710403200202

Blitz, L. V., Anderson, E. M., & Saastamoinen, M. (2016). Assessing perceptions of culture and trauma in an elementary school: Informing a model for culturally responsive trauma-informed schools. *The Urban Review, 48*(4), 520–542. https://doi.org/10.1007/s11256-016-0366-9

De Vynck, E., Boynton, H. M., & Burns, V. F. (2023). Pulled from the shoreline in search of spacious spirituality: Journeys of spiritual distress, resilience, and posttraumatic growth for women of evangelical Christian backgrounds in a Canadian context. *Religions, 14*, 1193. https://doi.org/10.3390/rel14091193

Doyle, T. P. (2009). The spiritual trauma experienced by victims of sexual abuse by Catholic clergy. *Pastoral Psychology, 58*, 239–260.

Duffell, N., & Basset, T. (2016). *Trauma, abandonment and privilege*. Routledge.

Ellis, H. M., Hook, J. N., Freund, C., Kranendonk, J., Zuniga, S., Davis, D. E., & Van Tongeren, D. R. (2023). *Religious/spiritual abuse and psychological and spiritual functioning.* Spirituality in Clinical Practice. https://psychnet.apa.org/record/2024-16105-001. https://doi.org/10.1037/scp0000346

Flynn, K. (2008). In their own voices: Women who were sexually abused by members of the clergy. *Journal of Child Sexual Abuse, 17*, 216–237.

Harris, R. (2002). *Christ-centred therapy: Empowering the self.* Routledge.

Herman, J. (2015). *Trauma and recovery. The aftermath of violence from domestic abuse to political terror*. Basic Books.

Heyder, R. (2022). Narrating and remembrance in the face of abuse in the church. *Religions, 13*, 348.

Jenkinson, G. (2008). An investigation into cult pseudo-personality: What is it and how does it form? *Cultic Studies Review, 7*(3), 199–224.

Jenkinson, G. (2019a, March). Out in the world: Post-cult recovery. *Therapy Today*, pp. 23–26.

Jenkinson, G. (2019b). *Post-cult counselling workbook. A guide for your recovery and growth.* Hope Valley Counselling.

Koenig, H. G., & Larson, D. B. (2001). Religion and mental health: Evidence for an association. *International Review of Psychiatry, 13*, 67–78. https://doi.org/10.1080/09540260124661

Kübler-Ross, E. (1969). *On death and dying.* (40th anniversary ed.). Routledge.

Kübler-Ross, E., & Kessler, D. (2005). *On grief and grieving: Finding the meaning of grief through the five stages of loss.* Scribner.

Lifton, R. J. (1989). *Thought reform and the psychology of totalism. A study of "brainwashing" in China.* University of North Carolina Press.

Marich, J. (2024). *You lied to me about God.* North Atlantic Books.

Mathis-Rimes, C. (2018). *Cruel sanctuary: A young woman's battle to escape from a fanatical religious sect.* Amazon.

McConnaughey, J. (2022). *Trauma in the pews. The impact on faith and spiritual practices.* Berry Powell Press.

Mearns, D., & Thorne, B. (2007). *Person-centred counselling in action.* Sage.

Mearns, D., & Thorne, B., with McCleod, J. (2013). *Person-centred counselling in action* (4th ed.). Sage.

Nica, A. (2019). Exiters of religious fundamentalism: Reconstruction of social support and relationships related to well-being. *Mental Health, Religion & Culture, 22*(5), 543–556. https://doi.org/10.1080/13674676.2019.1636015

Oakley, L., & Humphreys, J. (2019). *Escaping the maze of spiritual abuse.* Society for Promoting Christian Knowledge.

Pargament, K. I., Murray-Swank, N. A., & Mahoney, A. (2008). Problem and solution: The spiritual dimension of clergy sexual abuse and its impact on survivors. *Journal of Child Sexual Abuse, 17*, 397–420.

Perry, S. (2024). Religious/spiritual abuse, meaning-making and posttraumatic growth. *Religions, 15*(824), 1–10. https://doi.org/10.3390/rel15070824

Rogers, C. R. (1961). *On becoming a person. A therapist's view of psychotherapy.* Houghton Mifflin.

Rogers, F. (2024). Spiritual dimensions of trauma and posttraumatic growth: An ethnographic exploration. *Religions, 15*(926), 1–10. https://doi.org/10.3390/rel15080926

Roudkovski, K. (2024). *Understanding spiritual abuse. What it is and how to respond.* B&H Academic.

Shonkoff, J., & Garner, A. (2012). The committee on psychosocial aspects of child and family health, committee on early childhood adoption and dependent care, and section on developmental and behavioral pediatrics. *Pediatrics, 129*(1), 232–246.

Singer, M. T. (2003). *Cults in our midst: The continuing fight against their hidden menace.* Jossey-Bass.

Vazquez, V. E., Pate, R. A., MacCullum, J., Matta, M., Zivanovic, S., Chamberlin, S., Baker, T., & Newman, S. (2022). Deliberate rumination and posttraumatic growth: The mediating role of Christian gratitude and attachment to God. *Mental Health, Religion & Culture, 25*(8), 755–773. https://doi.org/10.1080/13674676.2022.2102160

Vis, J.-A.A., & Boynton, H. M. (2008). Spirituality and transcendent meaning making: Possibilities for enhancing posttraumatic growth. *Journal of Religion and Spirituality in Social Work: Social Thought, 27*, 69–86.

Waite, R., & Ryan, R. A. (2020). *Adverse childhood experiences.* Routledge.

Winnicott, D. W. (1965). A clinical study of the effect of a failure of the average expectable environment on a child's mental functioning. *The International Journal of Psycho-Analysis, 46*, 81.

Wortmann, J. H., & Park, C. L. (2008). Religion/spirituality in adjustment following bereavement: An integrative review. *Death Studies, 32*, 703–736. https://doi.org/10.1080/07481180802289507

Yalom, I. D. (2017). *Becoming myself. A psychiatrist's memoir.* Little, Brown.

Zieman, B. (2017). *Cracking the cult code for therapists. What every cult victim wants their therapist to know.* CreateSpace Independent Publishing Platform.

Zieman, B. (2018) *Shunned: A survival guide.* Amazon.

10

Implications for Counsellors, Psychotherapists, and Other Related Professionals

Introduction

The focus of this chapter and the next will be on the literature and research findings for professionals. While mainly written for counselling and psychotherapy practitioners, they will also apply to the work of spiritual direction, chaplaincy, coaching, pastoral care, and social work.

Eva and Anna acknowledged the importance of the counsellor's understanding. Francesca Alexandra said that a therapist who was highly attuned and who understood and soothed her was crucial to her healing. Hannah shared that she once had a non-Jewish therapist who was just not following the conversation, so she could not continue with them, but then had a Jewish counsellor with a different level of observance and background to her, but who she felt understood her. For Maya, her twice-weekly therapy and participation in this research were helpful.

For practitioners, the issue of the most effective theoretical approach to use when working with religious abuse survivors is crucial, but the literature on this is sparse because members of high-demand groups are discouraged from seeking psychological input. The next section explores *some* of the possible theoretical approaches that might be used.

G. Harvey, *Fundamentalist Religious Childhoods and Adult Mental Health and Wellbeing*, https://doi.org/10.1007/978-3-032-20140-9_10

Person-Centred Therapy (PCT)

The question is whether the person-centred perspective with the therapeutic alliance, the core conditions (Rogers, 1961), and narrative at heart are necessary and sufficient for religious trauma clients. Being client-led and narrative in nature, driven by philosophical conviction, the bottom layer of Bond's Pond (Bond, 1995, cited in Palmer & Woolfe, 2000) is that all clients, including traumatised ones, have an actualising tendency and an organismic self. This can facilitate an immense capacity to heal, given the provision of a 'growth producing climate' (Mearns & Thorne, 2013, p. 13). The skills used, the top layer of Bond's Pond (Bond, 1995, cited in Palmer & Woolfe, 2000), are conveyance of the core conditions (Rogers, 1961) through active listening, such as making appropriate eye contact, reflecting, clarifying, paraphrasing, and summarising. 'The relationship is core to the therapy' (Knox & Cooper, 2015, p. ix); this is important because 'the therapeutic relationship is the cornerstone of all effective treatment' (Van Der Kolk, 2003, cited in Carey, 2006, p. 17). Containment for religious trauma for clients who have experienced betrayal of trust means that the sanctity of the therapeutic space can create 'a slow and gentle approach while the therapist maintains a calm but caring attitude' (Murray Parks & Prigerson, 2010 p. 157).

The efficacy of person-centred therapy (Rogers, 1959) is barely covered in the trauma literature, with this modality viewed as lacking the knowledge and skills to work with complex trauma (Joseph, 2015), although another perspective is that the philosophy behind Rogers' (1959) work is consistent with trauma theory. One view is that while this supportive therapy might be helpful to well-adjusted clients seeking to deal with trauma, it is unlikely to offer appropriate interventions for those who have complex trauma (Mavranezouli et al., 2020). Conversely, Bullock (2020) asserts that a non-directive person-centred approach can be latrogenic when working with trauma survivors, with some critics insisting that specialist training is required to work with complex trauma (de Thierry, 2018).

One suggestion is that the therapeutic relationship, which lies at the heart of the person-centred approach, is far more important than the specific modality (Norcross and Wampold (2019), with Schwartz (2020,

p. 2) asserting that healing from complex PTSD 'often requires a positive relationship with a therapist who fully accepts you for who you are and helps you to reclaim your trust in other people'. This is an important consideration strengthened by meta-analysis outcomes (Norcross & Wampold, 2019), which show that the therapeutic relationship plays a key part in the reduction of symptoms for traumatised clients. The American Psychological Association (APA) (2011) recognises the importance of the therapeutic bond to recovery. Being listened to and heard are important to healing (Bashant, 2021), as is being in a safe therapeutic relationship (Briere & Scott, 2015; Ellinghaus et al., 2020). However, many clients who have grown up in a strict religious setting will be reluctant to build a therapeutic alliance, having been taught to prefer 'faith-based methods of treatment' (Friedson, 2015, p. 693). Other barriers to therapeutic connection are that JWs and other fundamentalist religions teach their members not to trust or develop intimate relationships with outsiders. Interestingly, the UK National Institute for Clinical Excellence (NICE) guidelines (2005) for PTSD list 'supportive counselling: NICE's definition of person centred counselling' (Reeves, 2013, pp. 206–207) as appropriate treatment. The person-centred (PC) approach does not have the monopoly on safe, therapeutic relationships; however, as this may also be an important part of other theoretical orientations, such as Jenkinson's (2019) relational, psycho-educative model.

Cognitive Behavioural Therapy (CBT)

There are those researchers, mainly of a cognitive behavioural orientation, who argue that some therapies, mainly cognitive behavioural ones are more efficacious for certain forms of psychological distress than others (Chambless, 2002; Hunsley & Di Giulio, 2002, cited in Cooper, 2008, p. 36).

Conversely, there are researchers, mainly from non-cognitive behavioural therapy backgrounds, who argue that the different therapies are similar in their overall efficacy (Assay & Lambert, 1999; 2002 cited in Cooper, 2008). However, CBT has been shown to effectively help lessen the symptoms of PTSD, 'with clinical improvement rates of around 50 per cent for clients traumatised by rape, assault and war' (Bradley et al., 2005, cited in Cooper, 2008, p. 40). Yet, CBT is often criticised for ignoring the importance of the therapeutic relationship. The need for a good therapeutic alliance, regardless of the theoretical modality of the therapist, is backed by research evidence which showed that 'relational factors account(ed) for around 30 per cent of the variance in outcomes' (Assay & Lambert, 1999, cited in Cooper, 2008, p. 99). It was the characteristics that differed, since it was collaborative with the focus on symptoms, rather than the narrative, the aim being to 'attempt to change the problematic meanings of the traumatic experience' (Joseph, 2015, p. 3). Roudkovski (2024) claims that cognitive processing therapy (CPT), which focuses on trauma-associated thoughts, is a research-validated, efficacious treatment for the processing of trauma and reducing the symptoms of PTSD. The statistical evidence in favour of CBT-type therapies as treatment for religious trauma can be attributed to its measurability, in contrast to PC work, since the evidence for its efficacy is largely anecdotal.

Yet, the National Institute for Health and Care Excellence (NICE) (2018)recommended CBT as a preferred treatment method for PTSD. The outcomes of meta-analysis research revealed strong indications of the efficacy of these treatments for single-event trauma for adults (Lancaster et al., 2016) and young people (Mavranezouli et al., 2020). Further evidence showing that these treatments can effectively treat complex trauma across populaces National Institute for Health and Care Research (NIHR) (2021), although all studies recognise that more quality evidence of outcomes is required.

The leading discursive discourse is that CBT has been afforded political, cultural, and therapeutic dominance in recent times, backed by government investment that has secured the treatment of mental health issues in the UK (Williams, 2015). The accusation is that a therapeutic monopoly exists. While meta-analyses utilising randomised control trials (RCT) have shown that Trauma Focused-CBT (TF-CBT), which integrates some psycho-educative interventions such as coping techniques, graded exposure, and cognitive rationalisation, can effectively reduce symptoms suggestive of complex trauma (de Arellano et al., 2014), the argument that CBT has been well marketed but is ineffective in the treatment of complex traumatic experiences is persuasive. Yet, Hiller et al. (2021) argue that the findings of their longitudinal study eradicate such criticism, and Gillies et al. (2016) pinpoint the need for research that compares the effectiveness of the different psychological therapies for treating complex trauma. The domination of RCTs in current research findings on this topic is criticised for being limited in application (McLeod, 2019). Research into the effectiveness of other therapeutic modalities is noticeably absent, and there is little understanding of their strengths and weaknesses (Mavranezouli et al., 2020), although this does not necessarily mean that they are ineffective (Joseph, 2004). The most studied approach, CBT, is not necessarily the most effective (Norcross & Wampold, 2019). However, it has been listed in the UK NICE guidelines (NICE, 2005) as an effective treatment for traumatic experiences (Reeves, 2013).

Eye movement Desensitisation and Reprocessing (EMDR)

EMDR is also highly researched and may be an efficacious way of healing religious trauma through its eight-phase therapeutic model. The arguable beneficial aspect of EMDR is that the client does not need to re-tell their story with the inherent danger of re-traumatisation, yet survivors often report the benefits of retelling their story as part of healing (Roudkovski, 2024). The downside of EMDR is that it is expensive for the client and practitioner, with several weekly sessions needed for the client and extensive specialist further practitioner training necessitated.

Psychodynamic Therapy

This approach 'engag(es) the individual in a process wherein the unconscious is the main avenue toward exploration' (Friedson, 2015, p. 694). The examination of the past and the nature of early associations are also investigated in attempting to understand the client's later relationships. Many other factors are integral to this form of therapy, including:

> … mirroring and validating patients' experiences, helping them to articulate a core life narrative, containing painful affect that might otherwise become overwhelming, bearing witness to that pain and facilitating an emotional experience that is reparative because it is in some way different from previous experiences that felt disappointing, misattuned or painful. (Friedson, 2015, p. 694)

Psychodynamic therapy recognises the unconscious transference processes that often exist. The binary nature of the strict religious environment can lead to the client 'splitting', seeing the therapist as 'either all good or all bad' (Friedson, 2015, p. 708). At the crux of psychotherapy lies exploration, questioning, and the client being open to challenge. This can be significantly difficult for someone who has grown up in an environment where restrictions meant these were harshly prohibited. It is noteworthy that 'psycho-dynamically orientated therapists tend to take an interest in treating individuals in an integrated way' (Friedson, 2015, p. 708).

An Integrative Approach

An integrative approach, which incorporates the relational aspects of the person-centred approach with psychoeducation and embodiment, can be beneficial for some people. The Gestalt concept of introjects, the drama triangle and the parent, adult, child model of Transactional Analysis, the focus on thinking and behaviour of CBT or CPT, together with the window of tolerance of sensorimotor psychotherapy (Ogden et al., 2006) and polyvagal theory (Porges, 2017) are examples of what might be helpful to the client in helping them to understand their trauma reactions.

There is currently no one training path to becoming competent in working with religious abuse survivors. While this is a contentious issue, Roudkovski (2024, p. 152) convincingly differentiates between therapeutic methods that primarily have a 'top-down' (changing thoughts and behaviours), or 'bottom-up approach' (working with the trauma stored in the body). Rationalising her preference for the latter, she states that strategies such as deep breathing and sensorimotor actions can be beneficial for a survivor of spiritual abuse.

Please note that the case studies presented are an amalgam of clients that I have worked with over the years. Some details have been changed to protect confidentiality and anonymity.

Case Study 1: Susan

Susan was allocated up to twenty sessions funded by the redress scheme for the strict Christian group that her family were multi-generationally involved in. She told me when I first met her that she was married with three primary school-aged children and worked in a Christian church as an outreach worker. She was struggling with her work setting because she no longer had any religious beliefs or practices.

She was not compliant in her growing-up years and told me that she rebelled against being told what to do, the restrictions she experienced, and having to be well-behaved at the very long meetings she was forced to attend. She described how she was humiliated for non-compliance and carried out of meetings as physical punishment for wriggling in her seat. She also related how the children from the group were forced to go home from school for lunch so that they were not influenced by their 'worldly' peers in the playground.

Susan was resistant to forming a therapeutic bond in the early stages because she had been taught not to trust outsiders. She also struggled to believe that psychotherapy could help her change.

Reflective questions If client Susan came to you for counselling, what therapeutic approach/es would you use?

Do you believe that you could work ethically and knowledgeably, given her strict religious upbringing?

How might you acknowledge her resistance to believing that therapy might be helpful?

Ethical Working with Survivors of Developmental Religious Abuse

> Ethics is a discipline within philosophy that is concerned with human contact and moral decision making. (Remley & Herlihy, 2001, p. 2)

All those working in the caring professions must seek to adhere to the relevant ethical code. The UK counselling and psychotherapy professional bodies, including the British Association for Counselling and Psychotherapy (BACP), the Association of Christians in Counselling and Linked Professions (ACC), the UK Council for Psychotherapy, and the National Counselling and Psychotherapy Society (NCPS), all have such guidelines. While Harborne (2012) argued that psychotherapy and spiritual direction were identical except that the former prioritised boundaries, contracts, and supervision, at that time, spiritual direction lacked them. This has changed since, with the London Centre for Spiritual Direction (LCSD), The Retreat Association UK, and Spiritual Direction International all having ethical guidelines now. This is crucial, as it is a directee-director relationship of safety and trust where love dwells and where the 'special and sacred identity' (O'Donohue, 1997, p. 36) of each person 'can bring the gift of presence and light, graced by affection'. The ethical principles of beneficence as 'a commitment to promoting the client's well-being' (BACP Ethical Framework, 2018, p. 3) and non-maleficence as 'a commitment to avoiding harm to the client' (BACP Ethical Framework, 2018, p. 3) must be a priority for all caring professionals.

The Inclusion of Religion/Spirituality in the Therapeutic Space

While spiritual directors, pastoral carers, and chaplains openly work with religious matters, therapy has historically been viewed as a secular practice without the inclusion of religion. Hansen (1998) acknowledges that the influence of childhood religion on development is often overlooked in counselling and psychotherapy, while Miller's (1999) perspective is that the importance of religion/spirituality in counselling has long been recognised. While the former is true in the UK, the opposite is the case in the USA, where, in line with the burgeoning interest in religion and health, the importance of religion/spirituality to some counselling clients has increasingly been attended to by the Council for Accreditation of Counselling and Related Educational Programs (CACREP) (2016), the American Counselling Association (ACA) Ethical Code, and the Association for Spiritual, Ethical, and Religious Values in Counselling (ASERVIC) Spiritual Competencies (2009). The need for counsellors to be trained to work with the religious/spiritual worldviews of clients and to recognise the influence of their own biases on the therapeutic work is the reason why religion/spirituality is now included in the syllabus of many US training programmes (Cashwell & Young, 2004; Parker, 2009).

In the UK, findings have indicated that counsellors can feel ill-equipped to work with such matters and would like further training in this area (Christodoulidi, 2011; Hofmann & Walach, 2011). This need was highlighted in one UK heuristic Interpretative Phenomenological Analysis (IPA) study of five counsellors, none of whom had received any training on working with visceral or vicarious trauma or spirituality, apart from one US participant (Gubi & Jacobs, 2009). Within the UK psychotherapy profession, there were only American competency frameworks for working with matters of religion and spirituality until the launch of 'The Churchill Framework' (Churchill, 2021). This provides a competency framework for counsellors working with their clients' religious/spiritual issues, and guidelines for working with them. While the origins are Christian, the claim is that it can also be utilised when working with clients from different religious traditions. This assertion may be overambitious because the author identifies as Christian, so the inherent conscious and unconscious biases (Guccione & Wellington, 2017) that one religious worldview brings may prevent it from being more widely applicable. However, this development is to be welcomed, given that guidelines are provided for working with religion and spirituality. Many of the guidelines are relevant to the research topic, in recognition of both the benefits and the shadow side of a fundamentalist religious childhood on wellbeing in later life. These include the offering of respect, acceptance, and non-judgementalism (A3), the development of a self-critical and reflective approach (C6), and the important role of supervision (D1, D2, D3, D4) in supporting ethical and professional 'trauma-informed' (Cashwell & Swindle, 2018, p. 182; Treisman, 2021) client work and supervisee wellbeing, bearing in mind the possibility of vicarious trauma (Rothschild, 2006; Williams et al., 2012). In acknowledgement of the beneficial and detrimental effects of religion on psychosocial functioning and the emotive nature of religious and spiritual matters (Swindle, 2017), Cashwell and Swindle (2018) highlight the importance of attending to the supervisory relationship and the supervisee's needs and emotions, encouraging supervisees to reflect on their own religious beliefs and experiences, assessment of the counsellor's tolerance levels and susceptibilities, issues of transference and countertransference, supporting the supervisee by appropriately bracketing off their own experiences, and enabling counsellors to present such matters. This paper originates in the USA and conceptualises religious abuse as being perpetrated by leaders within religious communities, and fails to account for occurrences within family settings, a much-neglected area within psychotherapy (Novšak et al., 2012). The need for informed practice is demonstrated in Gubi and Jacobs' (2009) discovery that four out of five participants self-reported traumatisation by working with spiritually abused clients, but it was challenging to find a supervisor who could work with spiritual issues, with counsellors experiencing mixed proficiency in the supervisory environment.

Kinmond et al. (2019) acknowledge the lack of research and direction for working with child abuse linked to faith or belief (CALFB) within the UK literature and the paucity of attention paid to this within the UK counselling profession, despite the likelihood of this presenting. As part of a wider study, they carried out an online survey, with 79 of the participants identifying as counsellors. The outcomes were that while 79 per cent had encountered the term CALFB, only 54 per cent felt they could respond with assurance. While many of the therapists were interested in developing their competencies to work with CALFB, only 34 per cent had received specialist training. This resonates with the findings of the wider mixed methods online survey of 1,361 contributors (Oakley et al., 2019) that revealed a convincing need for 'frontline practitioners' to become faith-literate about both the benefits and abusive effects of religiously related child abuse. The multidimensional nature of childhood religious abuse, which the literature shows has often been disguised and validated (Novšak et al., 2012) as acceptable, means that the detrimental effects can present in the therapeutic space at the individual, inter-relational, systemic, and spiritual levels. Leighton (2014, p. 298) says that clients who hold rigid, dogmatic, and literal religious beliefs may view counselling as 'the handiwork of the devil', and stresses the importance of rigorous assessment procedures and the building of the therapeutic relationship.

> To heal the world, we must first heal ourselves, and that likely needs to include an exploration of our spiritual and religious history so that we can heal its wounds that are still vulnerably tender. (Marich, 2024, p. 20)

Trauma-Informed Practice

Many theoretical frameworks and strategies can be used when working with the complexity of presentation with religious trauma survivors. All of the co-researchers voiced the importance of therapists working in a trauma-informed way (Cashwell & Swindle, 2018; Treisman, 2021). The literature also emphasises the significance of working in this way (Roudkovski, 2024; Swindle et al., 2024), which involves being aware of the multiple ways in which a person can be impacted biologically, psychologically, socially, and neurologically (Swindle et al., 2024). The presenting issue is not problematised or diagnosed, but instead the counsellor seeks to understand what has happened to the client in line with the power threat meaning framework (Boyle & Johnstone, 2020).

An understanding of neuroscience can be an integral part of trauma work because 'the development of neuropsychology has provided further insight into how and why traumatic memory differs from non-traumatic memory' (Reeves, 2013, p. 204). It can also be helpful to understand that distortion around memory is common in that 'sometimes a traumatic event is completely forgotten. Often the incident is remembered, though incompletely or in fragments' (Rothschild, 2011, p. 41). One research study by Rauch et al. (1996) played two audiotapes to eight subjects. One tape was neutral, and the other one related a traumatic event with the subjects' heart rates and regional cerebral blood flow (RCBF) measured via positron emission tomography (PET) scans. In the areas of the brain thought to be involved with intense emotion, the RCBF was greater when listening to the traumatic audiotape than the neutral one. In contrast, 'there was a decrease in RCBF in and around Broca's area' (cited in Cozolino, 2010, p. 275) 'an area of the interior frontal cortex that controls speech'. The importance of reactivating Broca's area of the brain through narrative and reassuring a client that they are remembering a terrible experience that happened many years ago can be key. The therapist supporting the client in understanding that it is a memory and not happening in the present (Cozolino, 2010, p. 277) can be a crucial part of trauma-informed therapy.

This is important because what keeps trauma stuck is that the survivor has been unable to relocate the memories in the past. The result of this is that 'a survivor's amygdalae continue to react as if the traumatic threat persists, provoking the autonomic nervous system to attain the state of fight, flight, or freeze–whichever was activated at the original time of the trauma' (Rothschild, 2011, p. 41). Trauma is so difficult to define and understand because it 'is not the event itself; rather, trauma resides in the nervous system' (Levine & Kline, 2007, p. 4).

Trauma-informed practice also means that the practitioner will keep in mind the possibility of re-traumatisation, which is when a client 'experiences the same level of distress as during the original trauma' (Reeves, 2013, p. 2006) when working with memories. So while the processing of traumatic memories is common (Rothschild, 2011, p. 41), the debate is whether this is useful, given the argument that some clients 'soon become disabled by the practice. One perspective is that 'remembering is not required' (Rothschild, 2011, p. 41), and it is more beneficial to focus on the impact.

Yet, Roudkovski's (2024) perspective is that many survivors need to tell their story, with McBride (2025, loc 179) stressing the importance of this:

> Our wounds, whatever they are, are made more powerful by the silence around them. The naming of what has hurt us, how we have hurt others, and how these hurts still linger is the very undoing of the cloak that keeps the pain unseen and unaddressed. And this – the naming, the unveiling, the unsettling – as painful as it is, is central to how we heal.

There is evidence to show that 'the brain continues to reorganise itself by forming new neural connections throughout life' (Gergen, 2015, p. 15), facilitated by 'talking through the trauma with supportive others (which) creates the neuro-biological conditions for the reestablishment of neural coherence' (Cozolino, 2010, p. 263). This perspective is strengthened by the neuroscientific evidence regarding neural network integration and the importance of reactivating Broca's area of the brain inhibited in trauma. The problem is that there is not one clear evidence-based way of working with trauma generally and the effects of religious abuse specifically. 'Psychotherapy is not medicine, and the human psyche has many, many variables' (Rothschild, 2011, p. 65). While CBT is based on outcome research, in that measurements are used at the beginning, middle, and end to evaluate progress, many other psychotherapy approaches produce anecdotal rather than quantifiable results, but that may not matter.

There is not one preferred modality, but working in a bespoke way while keeping the ethical guidelines in mind is essential. Guidance such as that issued by the British Psychological Society (BPS) on working with recovered memories can be useful, as it reminds both client and practitioner to tolerate uncertainty in the work (Bond, 2015). The importance of pacing the work is also crucial: 'Levine likens it to having a foot on the accelerator and brake at the same time' (Lee Cori, 2007, p. 15).

Working in a trauma-informed way also means utilising a model for recovery, such as a three-phase approach with 'phase I being stabilisation and safety, phase II remembering and processing trauma memories and phase III integration with family, culture and normal daily life' (Janet, 1898/1919, cited in Rothschild, 2011, p. 57). Miller (2023, p. 118) claims that, based on Herman's trauma recovery stages of establishing safety, remembrance and mourning, and re-connection, she has developed a five-stage model for religious trauma recovery:

deconstruction (addressing cognitive dissonance);
safety and autonomy (creating a lifestyle of psychological safety);
remembrance and reframing (telling and validating your story);
self-understanding (getting to know yourself authentically;
healthy relationships (reimagining how to relate to others).

All trauma recovery models assert that creating stabilisation and safety before the survivor tells their story is crucially important. Stages models are frequently critiqued for suggesting a progressive path to healing; however, they can be helpful to realise that working towards healing commonly involves many oscillations between all of the phases, with grounding techniques sometimes being triggering for clients. The first stage of trauma recovery aims to help the client self-regulate using grounding techniques such as breathing exercises and mindfulness. This is crucially important, otherwise 'it's like sending a car down a slippery hill with no brakes' (Lee Cori, 2007, p. 108). Trauma resides in 'the unspoken voice' (Levine, 2010, p. 9) and can manifest in a wide variety of physical symptoms. Sometimes clients physically shake as they talk about traumatic events, and the importance of this has been recognised: 'the shaking and trembling … are a core part of the innate process that resets my nervous system and helps to restore my psyche to wholeness' (Levine, 2010, p. 15). When this happens, being wrapped (with permission) or the client wrapping themselves in a blanket to help self-regulation can be helpful because 'in order to put the past in the past, clients must process traumatic experiences in the optimal arousal zone' (Wilbarger & Wilbarger, 1997, cited in Ogden et al., 2006, p. 27). This is where psychoeducation about the window of tolerance might be helpful because, until safety and stabilisation are accessible, re-traumatisation can happen.

The cognitive process of deconstruction is conceptualised as the first stage of religious trauma recovery, being cognitive and therefore potentially less triggering. Deconstruction has been defined as:

> ... a process of breaking down and analysing the various parts of a belief system and its practices. (Miller, 2023, p. 125)

This involves the client moving from the rigidity of a fundamentalist belief system into 'cognitive flexibility' (Miller, 2023, p. 126), tolerating uncertainty while also learning to critique and question, maybe for the first time. The next chapter will consider how professionals can facilitate client recovery from religious trauma and how survivors might present in the therapeutic space. Case studies will also be provided, together with thought-provoking questions for professionals to reflect on.

References

American Psychiatric Association. (2011). *Diagnostic and statistical manual of mental disorders* (5th ed.). American Psychiatric Association.

Association for Spiritual, Ethical and Religious Values in Counselling. (2009). *Spiritual competences: Competences for addressing spiritual and religious issues in counseling.* Retrieved March 31 2018, from http://www.aservic.org/wp-content/uploads/2018/03/Spiritual-Competencies-Printer-friendly1.pdf

Council for Accreditation of Counseling and Related Educational Programs. (2016). *2016 CACREP standards.* Retrieved March 7, 2016, from https://www.cacrep.org/wp-content/uploads/2016/02/2016-Standards-with-Glossary-rev2.2016.pdf

Bashant, J. (2021,15 June). *Anxiety, trauma & self-harm in children and adolescents—Essential regulation and restorative practices.* [Live webcast]. PESI training. https://www.pesi.co.uk

Bond, T. (2015). *Standards and ethics for counselling in action* (4th ed). Sage.

Boyle, M., & Johnstone, L. (2020). *A straight talking introduction to the power threat meaning framework: An alternative to psychiatric diagnosis.* PCCS Books.

Briere, J., & Scott, C. (2015). Complex trauma in adolescents and adults: Effects and treatment. *The Psychiatric Clinics of North America, 28*(3). https://doi.org/10.1016/j.psc.2015.05.004

British Association for Counselling and Psychotherapy. (2018). *Ethical framework for the counselling professions.* BACP.

Bullock, P. (2020). Is counselling enough to treat trauma? *Therapy Today, 31*(3), 31–33.

Carey, L. (2006). *Expressive and creative arts methods for trauma survivors.* Jessica Kingsley.

Cashwell, C. S., & Swindle, P. J. (2018). When religion hurts: Supervising cases of religious abuse. *The Clinical Supervisor, 37*(1), 182–203. https://doi.org/10.1080/07325223.2018.1443305

Cashwell, C. S., & Young, J. S. (2004). Spirituality in counsellor training: A content analysis of syllabi from introductory spirituality courses. *Counseling and Values, 48*, 96–109. https://doi.org/10.1002/j.2161-007X.2004.tb00237.x

Christodoulidi, F. (2011). Counselling, spirituality, and culture. In W. West (Ed.), *Exploring therapy, spirituality and healing.* Palgrave Macmillan.

Churchill, H. (2021). The Churchill Framework: A core-competence framework when working with clients' religious/spiritual issues in clinical practice. *Accord, 110*(Spring), 21–27.

Cooper, M. (2008). *Essential research findings in counselling and psychotherapy: The facts are friendly.* Sage.

Cozolino, L. (2010). *The neuroscience of psychotherapy. Healing the social brain* (2nd ed.). W. W. Norton.

de Arellano, M., Lyman, D., Jobe-Shields, L., George, P., Dougherty, R., Daniels, A., Ghose, S., Huang, L., & Delphin-Rittmon, M. (2014). Trauma-focused cognitive-behavioural for children and adolescents: Assessing the evidence? *Psychiatric Services, 65*(5), 591–602. https://doi.org/10.1176/appi.ps.201300255

de Thierry, B. (2018). Recovery from trauma not management of behaviour. *BACP Children, Young People and Families.* https://www.bacp.co.uk/bacp-journals/bacp-children-young-people-and-families-journal/september-2018/recovery-from-trauma/

Ellinghaus, C., Truss, K., Siling, J. L., Phillips, L., Eastwood, O., Medrano, C., & Bendall, S. (2020). I'm tired of being pulled from pillar to post:

A qualitative analysis of barriers to mental health care for trauma-exposed young people. *Early Intervention in Psychiatry, 15*(1), 113–122. https://doi.org/10.1111/eip.12919

Friedson, M. L. (2015). Psychotherapy and the fundamentalist client: The aims and challenges of treating Jehovah's Witnesses. *Journal of Religious Health, 54*, 693–712. https://doi.org/10.1007/s10943-014-9946-8

Gergen, K. J. (2015). The limits of neuroscience. *Therapy Today, 26*(6), 12–17.

Gillies, D., Maiocchi, L., Bhandari, A. P., Taylor, F., Gray, C., & O'Brien, L. (2016). Psychological therapies for children and adolescents exposed to trauma. *The Cochrane Database of Systematic Reviews, 10*(10). https://doi.org/10.1002/14651858.CD012371

Gubi, P. M., & Jacobs, R. (2009). Exploring the impact on counsellors of working with spiritually abused clients. *Mental Health, Religion & Culture, 12*, 191–204. https://doi.org/10.1080/13674670802441509

Guccione, K., & Wellington, J. (2017). *Taking control of writing your thesis.* Bloomsbury Academic.

Hansen, C. (1998). Long-term effects of religious upbringing. *Mental Health, Religion & Culture, 1*(2), 91–111. 10.1080/13674679808406502

Harborne, L. (2012), *Psychotherapy and spiritual direction. Two languages, one voice.* Karnac Books.

Hiller, R. M., Meiser-Stedman, R., Elliott, E., Banting, R., & Halligan, S. L. (2021). A longitudinal study of cognitive predictors of (complex) post-traumatic stress in young people in out-of-home care. *Journal of Child Psychology and Psychiatry, 62*(1), 48–57. https://doi.org/10.1111/jc13232

Hofmann, L., & Walach, H. (2011). Spirituality and religiosity in psychotherapy—A representative survey among German psychotherapists. *Psychotherapy Research, 21*(2), 179–192.

Jenkinson, G. (2019). *Post-cult counselling workbook. A guide for your recovery and growth.* Hope Valley Counselling.

Joseph, S. (2015). A person-centred perspective on working with people who have experienced psychological trauma and helping them to move forward to posttraumatic growth. *Person-Centred and Experiential Psychotherapies, 14*(3), 178–190. https://doi.org/10.1080/14779757.2015.1043392

Joseph, S. (2004). Client-centred therapy, post-traumatic stress disorder and post-traumatic growth: Theoretical perspectives and practical implications. *Psychology and Psychotherapy Theory Research and Practice, 77*(1), 101–119. https://doi.org/10.1348/147608304322874281

Kinmond, K., Oakley, L., Humphreys, J., & Dioum, M. (2019). Child abuse linked to faith or belief: An important issue for counselling practice. *British*

Journal of Guidance and Counselling, 47(6), 659–668. https://doi.org/10.1080/03069885.2017.1370696

Knox, R., & Cooper, M. (2015). *The therapeutic relationship in counselling and psychotherapy*. Sage.

Lancaster, C. L., Teeters, J. B., Gros, D. F., & Back, S. E. (2016). Post-traumatic stress disorder: Overview of evidence-based assessment and treatment. *Journal of Clinical Medicine, 5*(11), 105. https://doi.org/10.3390/jcm5110105

Lee Cori, J. (2007). *Healing from trauma. A survivor's guide to understanding your symptoms and reclaiming your life.* Marlowe.

Leighton, T. J. (2014). The therapeutics of counselling religious clients: Intake and assessment. *International Journal of Mental Health Addiction, 12*, 295–311. https://doi.org/10.1007/s11469-013-9454-1

Levine, P. A. (2010). *In an unspoken voice: How the body releases trauma and restores goodness.* North Atlantic Books.

Levine, P. A., & Kline, M. (2007). *Trauma through a child's eyes*. North Atlantic Books.

Marich, J. (2024). *You lied to me about God.* North Atlantic Books.

Mavranezouli, I., Megnin-Viggars, Daly, C., Dias, S., Stockton, S., Meiser, S. R., Trickey, D., & Pilling, S. (2020). Research review: Psychological and psychosocial treatments for children and young people with post-traumatic stress disorder: A network meta-analysis. *Journal of Child Psychology and Psychiatry, 61*(1), 18–29. https://doi.org/10.1111/jc13094

McBride, H. L. (2025). *Holy hurt*. Brazos Press.

McLeod, J. (2019). Research: Where now? *Therapy Today, 30*(5), 42–43.

Mearns, D., & Thorne, B. (2013). *Person-centred counselling in action.* Sage.

Miller, A. C. (2023). *Religious trauma survival guide. Education and recovery tools for survivors and professionals.* Empathy Paradigm.

Miller, G. A. (1999). The development of the spiritual focus in counselling and counsellor education. *Journal of Counselling and Development, 77*, 498–501. https://doi.org/10.1002/j.1556-6676.1999.tb02478.x

Murray Parks, C., & Prigerson, H. G. (2010). *Bereavement, studies of grief in adult Life* (4th ed.). Penguin Books.

National Institute for Health Research. (2021). www.nihr.ac.uk

NICE Guidelines. (2005). https://www.nice.org.uk/guidance/

NICE Guidelines. (2018). https://www.nice.org.uk/guidance/

Norcross, J. C., & Wampold, B. E. (2019). Relationships and responsiveness in the psychological treatment of trauma: The tragedy of the APA Clinical

Practice Guideline. *Psychotherapy, 56*(3), 391–399. https://doi.org/10.1037/pst0000228

Novšak, R., Mandelj, T. R., & Simonič, B. (2012). Therapeutic implications of religious-related emotional abuse. *Journal of Aggression, Maltreatment and Trauma, 21*, 31–44. https://doi.org/10.1080/10926771.2011.627914

Oakley, L., Kinmond, K., Humphreys, J., & Dioum, M. (2019). Safeguarding children who are exposed to abuse linked to faith or belief. *Child Abuse Review, 28*, 27–38. https://doi.org/10.1002/car.2540

O'Donohue, J. (1997). *Anam cara. Spiritual wisdom from the Celtic world*. Bantam Books.

Ogden, P., Minton, K., & Pain, C. (2006). *Trauma and the body: A sensorimotor approach to psychotherapy*. Norton.

Palmer, A., & Woolfe, R. (2000). *Integrative and eclectic counselling and psychotherapy*. Sage.

Parker, S. (2009). Faith development theory as a context for supervision of spiritual and religious issues. *Counselor Education and Supervision, 49*(1), 39–53. https://doi.org/10.1002/j.1556-6978.2009.tb00085.x

Porges, S. W. (2017). *The pocket guide to the polyvagal theory: The transformative power of feeling safe*. Norton.

Rauch, S. L., Van der Kolk, B. A, Fisher, R. E. (1996). A symptom provocation study of posttraumatic stress disorder using positron emission tomography and script-driven imagery. *Arch Gen Psychiatry*, 53. 380–387.

Reeves, A. (2013). *An introduction to counselling and psychotherapy, from theory to practice*. Sage.

Remley, T. P., Jr., & Herlichy, B. (2001). *The handbook of counseling* (p. 69).

Rogers, C. R. (1961). *On becoming a person. A therapist's view of psychotherapy*. Houghton Mifflin.

Rogers, C. R. (1959). A theory of therapy, personality and interpersonal relationships, as developed in the client-centred framework. In S. Koch (Ed.), *Psychology: A study of science. 3 formulations of the person and the social* context (pp. 184–256). McGraw Hill.

Rothschild, B. (2011). *8 keys to safe trauma recovery: Take-charge strategies to empower your healing*. Norton.

Rothschild, B. with Rand, M. (2006). *Help for the helper: The psychophysiology of compassion fatigue and vicarious trauma*. W. W. Norton.

Roudkovski, K. (2024). *Understanding spiritual abuse. What it is and how to respond*. B&H Academic.

Schwartz, A. (2020). *A practical guide to complex PTSD: Compassion strategies to begin healing from childhood trauma*. Rockridge Press.

Swindle, P. J. (2017). *A twisting of the sacred: The lived experience of religious abuse.* PhD thesis, University of North Carolina. https://www.proquest.com/docview/1927630238?%20Theses&fromopenview=true&fromunauthdoc=true&pq-origsite=gscholar&sourcetype=Dissertations%20

Swindle, P. J., Cashwell, C., & Tangen, J. L. (2024). *Counseling survivors of religious abuse.* Routledge.

Treisman, K. (2021). *Trauma-inducing and trauma-reducing health and medical experiences drawing on stories from 390 people and some of the values of trauma-informed practice.* https://www.safehandsthinkingminds.co.uk

Williams, A., Helm, H. M., & Clemens, E. V. (2012). The effect of childhood trauma, personal wellness, supervisory working alliance, and organizational factors on vicarious traumatization. *Journal of Mental Health Counseling, 34*, 133–153. https://doi.org/10.17744/mehc.34.2.j3l62k872325h583

Williams, C. H. J. (2015). Improving access to psychological therapies and treatment outcomes: Epistemological assumptions and controversies. *Psychiatric and Mental Health Nursing, 22*(5), 344–351. https://doi.org/10.1111/jpm.12181

11
Further Implications

The Importance of Rigorous Assessment

Within the counselling and psychotherapy profession, there are many ways that an intake assessment is carried out, with multiple questions asked of the potential new client to avoid assumptions being made and to assess the feasibility of working together. Measurements, such as IES-R (Impact of Events Scale), GAD-7 (Anxiety), PHQ-9 (Depression), and PTSD scales, and also CORE forms, are sometimes used at the beginning and throughout the work.

Swindle et al. (2024) argue that there is a scarcity of tools available to assess religious harm, yet they identify the Religious Harm and Abuse Scale (RHAS), also known as the Spiritual Harm and Abuse Scale (SHAS) (Koch & Edstrom, 2024). This is a twenty-seven-item self-reporting list containing questions about 'lived experiences and emotional reactions' (Swindle et al., 2024, p. 39) but using only Christian terminology. Keller (2016) developed the Spiritual Abuse Questionnaire, which has seventeen statements aimed at those with previous or current involvement in churches. In response to the Christian nature of such religious harm assessment tools, Roudkovski (2024) developed an eleven-item inventory to assess for hurt in more diverse settings,

G. Harvey, *Fundamentalist Religious Childhoods and Adult Mental Health and Wellbeing*, https://doi.org/10.1007/978-3-032-20140-9_11

acknowledging that religious abuse happens in a variety of environments and relationships. An important part of the intake assessment considerations is that practitioners should be working within their levels of competency. Not all therapists would use measures and scores, as this relates to the theoretical modality, with a person-centred counsellor less likely to use them than a cognitive behavioural therapist.

It is important to emphasise that religious abuse may not be in the client's conscious awareness, as in the case study below. Measures and scores were not used at this intake assessment, but the terminology the client used to describe his birth parents alerted the therapist to the possibility of religious trauma.

Case Study 2: Martin

Martin came for counselling and had twelve sessions over seven months. In his mid-forties, he was very successful professionally, married with five children and had a strong Christian faith. His presenting issue was that he was struggling with his behaviour towards his wife, who had distanced herself for years. At the intake assessment, he described his mother as 'passionately Christian' and his father as 'very judgmental and an authoritarian narcissist'. Gradually, Martin explained that in his growing-up years, the home was 'a fortress', because although they were an extremely religious family, they did not attend church or Sunday school but operated 'like a cult' with his patriarchal father being 'the highest authority'. At the time, a person-centred approach seemed to be the best way of working, and he responded positively to the non-judgemental environment, empathy, unconditional positive regard, and genuineness, and started to put some 'loving distance' (Langone, 2016, cited in Aguado, 2018, p. 4) in place within previously enmeshed family relationships. During one session, I intuited that his internal dialogue was harsh and commented that I was not there to judge him. He was very tearful at that point and told me that he had felt judged all of his life. When ending counselling, he said that he had grown so much through counselling and yet, looking back now, I am left wondering whether I was in fact working with his cult pseudo-personality (Jenkinson, 2008) and wish that I had known then that a dysfunctional family can operate like a cult (Aguado, 2018).

Reflective Questions If Martin came to you for counselling, how would you work with him? Do you feel that you could work ethically and knowledgeably, given his strict religious upbringing, even though that was not the explicit presentation?

Might you be curious about this while acknowledging that the client had come to therapy because of his concern about his marital relationship?

Facilitating Client Recovery

As outlined in Chapter 10, an abundance of literature demonstrates that neuroscientific developments have enabled greater comprehension of the brain and its response to trauma (Fisher, 2017; van der Kolk, 2014). Modality integration is seen as valuable for trauma therapy, with more complex trauma requiring greater integration and flexibility viewed as crucial (Beck, 2020) to the avoidance of a mechanised 'one size fits all' approach (Fisher, 2017). Cooper (2008) asserts that while the therapeutic relationship is key to outcomes, therapists should not just do what they think is good. This is backed up by the American Psychiatric Association (2011), who state that unresearched treatments can be harmful to those who receive them. It is evident, then, that more research is needed around the psychological therapeutic combinations that are most effective, National Institute for Health and Care Research (NIHR) (2021).

Swindle (2017) argues that counsellors must recognise both the damaging and beneficial effects of clients' religious experiences, encouraging professionals to evaluate what aspects are useful for recovery and assess their support network. Zieman (2018) concurs and proposes techniques for calming the nervous system, as well as the development of an alternative social system for those who have exited their religious community. Psychoeducation might also assist recovery; for example, polyvagal theory (Porges, 2017), despite being criticised for its lack of empirical support, may help clients understand oscillations between the fight/flight zone (hyper-arousal) and freeze (hypo-arousal) and that functioning within these zones is a primal short-term survival mechanism. *When this becomes a more permanent 'modus operandi', it can be detrimental to health and wellbeing.*

One model suggests three stages of recovery: 'stage 1 – safety, stage 2 – remembrance and mourning, and stage 3 – reconnecting and meaning-making' (Herman, 2015, cited in Zieman, 2017, pp. 15–16). Jenkinson (2019b) developed a four-phase relational, psycho-educative approach to recovery, which recognises that progress is not linear (Jenkinson, 2019a) but that the client might oscillate between the stages. Knapp (2021) proposes a seven-stage model for optimum recovery from religious abuse and includes the provision of a constant metaphoric holding therapeutic environment. Novšak et al. (2012) agree that a multiple-stage process is needed, the first step being to understand the reality of the abusive experience. The purpose of therapy for religious abuse survivors is to look at their relational patterns and to recognise guilt, shame, and influential faith-based teachings, so that sessions can become a space for acknowledging personal responsibility, building new relationships, and facilitating healthy functioning.

The Misuse of Power and Control

One of the key findings from this study was power, control, and authoritarian fearmongering, as outlined in Chapter 7. Swindle et al., (2024, p. 35) name this as 'manipulation of the sacred to control' and provide examples such as pressurising members to stay in an abusive relationship, and using theology to manipulate and control members financially. Roudkovski (2024, pp. 89–96) states that control is gained by 'limiting personal agency, excessive accountability enforced by monitoring behaviour, performance-based acceptance, required obedience to the abuser, censuring and isolation'. Thought reform and brainwashing also play a part in the control of physical behaviour, the rational and emotional areas of functioning, and the information that members have access to. Anderson's religious power and control wheel visually illustrates that power and control lie at the heart of developmental religious abuse.

Reflective Questions How might counsellors facilitate client autonomy and address the inherent power imbalance in psychotherapy when working with religious trauma survivors?

Powerful Introjects

The Gestalt concept of introjects can be helpful in understanding that clients who have a strict religious background will have received many messages about beliefs, behaviours, and values and will have unconsciously 'swallowed whole' (Jenkinson, 2023, p. 91), unquestioned and unchallenged so that, like chewing gum, they sit in the gut unchewed is helpful to grasping this concept. Miller (2023, pp. 84–85) offers a 'developmental religious messages inventory' by listing some of the messages that religious groups explicitly teach or imply. These include 'I was born bad or sinful, God will only forgive me if I confess my sins, being influenced by non-believers is dangerous, and I should forgive anyone who hurts me' (Miller, 2023, p. 85). She also states that if a client ticks more than five of the thirty-six statements in the inventory, then there is a high likelihood that they suffered developmental religious trauma. The client may therefore present with at least some of these introjects as an integral part of their belief system, whether they have this awareness or not. Healing may involve bringing the introjects into conscious awareness and learning to challenge them.

Survivors of Religious Trauma/Spiritual Abuse Possible Presentations

Case Study 3: Robert

Robert is in his early twenties when he requests counselling. At the initial meeting, he stated that he grew up in a fundamentalist Christian church in which his whole family had been multi-generationally involved. He had started to question his faith as a teenager and no longer subscribed to the Christian beliefs that he was brought up with. However, he still lived in his parents' house as he could not afford to move out, and the Christian worship music that they regularly played was 'doing his head in'. He felt ashamed for playing his alternative music (very loudly) and having sex with his girlfriend in their house. Robert also felt very judged by his family for being an atheist, but struggled with his introjects: 'being angry is sinful and wrong, I should only have close relationships with other believers, and God will punish me by making bad things happen to me' (Miller, 2023, pp. 84–85).

> **Reflective Questions** What effect might the 'core conditions', especially unconditional positive regard in the therapeutic space, have on Robert?
> What might be some of the pros and cons of using a person-centred approach?

Shame and Perfectionism

A religious trauma client may present for psychotherapy with a strong sense of shame, whether they are aware of it or not. Weller (2015, p. 32) states:

> ... shame ruptures our connection with life and with our soul. It is, indeed, a sickness of the soul.

High-demand religious groups commonly have high standards and place huge responsibilities on members. Many members feel constantly ashamed and inadequate, trying to prove that they are 'good enough', while patterns of false guilt, unrealistic expectations, poor self-care, and excessive self-blame are their daily experiences. Notably, children who grow up in fundamentalist religious environments believe that they are bad and carry strong shame because they are unable to meet the high standards. Miller (2023, p. 27) asserts that:

> … this symptom is especially common in groups that teach that humans are fundamentally evil, sinful, or worthless on their own.

She also identifies 'self-criticism, self-neglect, learned helplessness, low self-trust, and purity shame' (Miller, 2023, pp. 27–28) as forms of it and states that a client might present in therapy with all or any of them.

Stressing the homogeneity requirements of high-demand religious environments, Friedson (2015) writes that a rupture of the therapeutic relationship might occur if the therapist asks questions, tries to explore alternative viewpoints, or challenges beliefs too quickly, taking into consideration that open exploration is often prohibited in fundamentalist religious settings. Friedson's (2015) perspective is that it might be advisable for a therapist to avoid questioning a client's deeply held religious beliefs. This agrees with the experience of an ex-member of a fundamentalist religious group who was instantly upset in a first session when the counsellor questioned her about her previous group's beliefs (McBeath & Greenlees, 2016). Another therapist has stated that her recovery only began when she started counselling with a therapist who understood the dynamics of a high-demand group (Jenkinson, 2013).

Case Study 4: Christine

Christine is a young married mother with two young children, who grew up in a high-control Christian group where the whole of her life was regulated by the group leaders. She was born into the group and described her lifestyle growing up as having benefits as well as difficulties.

While Christine and her family have since left the group, the introjects she swallowed whole as a child continue to be part of her internal dialogue, and she carries an enormous sense of guilt and shame while continuing to hold herself and others to high standards. She has found it difficult to adjust to the 'outside world' and to fit into a parent and toddler group. It soon becomes clear that she is highly self-critical, neglects herself, and fears being seen as proud.

Reflective Questions As a therapist, how might you handle Christine's need to see some of her upbringing as good?

Would you feel able to challenge her self-critical internal dialogue and neglect of self?

Chronic Fear and Anxiety Around Hell, Salvation, the Rapture, and Demons

In the research study, Francesca Alexandra described symptoms suggestive of C-PTSD. This is common for many religious trauma survivors who experience chronic anxiety symptoms such as general worries, panic attacks, nightmares, intrusive thoughts, and superstitious compulsions (Miller, 2023). Many fundamentalist religious groups teach about a conditional afterlife (heaven and hell), which can create great fear about burning forever. Karris (2023, p. xi) describes hell as 'a word packed with explosive imagery and fear-inducing meaning', the effects being on a continuum from mild to severe, and recognises the terror that such indoctrination creates. He recognises the existence of the Hell Anxiety Scale (Cranney et al., 2018), a questionnaire that can be used to measure the level of it, while acknowledging that the literature on this is sparse. 'Some Islamic beliefs about Johannam and the Fire (hell), are described as a place beneath the earth to eternally punish disbelievers and those who engage in other specified sins' (Thomassen, 2009, cited in Cole, 2023, p. 4). It is not surprising then that Karris (2023, p. 24) describes hell anxiety as 'a brutal form of psychological suffering that deserves attention'.

Other fears from Christianity include not being saved, being left behind at the rapture, and unseen, powerful supernatural forces that harm people. Miller (2023, pp. 35–36) helpfully indicates that the forms of fear and anxiety that religious trauma clients can suffer include 'after-life anxiety … supernatural anxiety, sexual dysfunction and religious cynicism' which she describes as 'difficulty feeling safe in religious settings due to suspicion, distrust, and paranoia about being controlled, exploited or manipulated by religious systems'.

Religious Scrupulosity

Fear and high anxiety can cause religious scrupulosity, a 'sub-type of [Obsessive Compulsive Disorder] (OCD) that literally means fearing sin where there is none' (Karris, 2023, p. 24). Drumsta (2023) similarly defines it as:

> … a condition that includes obsessions and compulsions, intrusive thoughts or urges with a religious theme. Often called Religious OCD.

One of the key characteristics is that religious behaviours and rituals are compulsively performed to offset high levels of anxiety, such as praying, reciting Bible verses, and writing down scripture repetitively, triggered by a huge fear of sinning and of God's punishment (Karris, 2023). Snyder (2023) shares her story of being consumed by her uncontrollable attempts to tolerate the uncertainty of relationships, sexuality, and faith. These compulsions were so great that her days were spent in prayer and confession, and nights were consumed by computer research while trying to understand her life experiences.

Case Study 5: John

John is a fifty-five-year-old client who describes himself as stuck in a prolonged bout of depression since the first COVID-19 lockdown, which resulted in the collapse of his business. At the assessment stage, he said that he completely lacked motivation, was awake all night and slept during the day, although he still felt 'sleep deprived'. He stated that he had been in almost continuous therapy for the previous two decades, including Cognitive Behavioural Therapy (CBT), general counselling, and longer-term psychotherapy where a 're-parenting approach' was taken. The longer-term work and one course of CBT had been the most helpful.

He related how, having become very ill as a child, he had developed a deep fear of death. He became a Christian as a result and was baptised into the faith in his teenage years. He had belonged to several churches over the years and was rejected for ministry training at one point. As a result, he had deconstructed his faith and no longer held any Christian beliefs. Yet, he was obsessively fearful of death and hell. He prayed compulsively and was terrified of dying in his sleep.

His mood was very low at assessment, although he was clear that he would never take his own life because of his fear of death and hell. John took many prescribed medications for his many physical ailments and his mental health challenges; however, he still felt hopeless and despairing.

Reflective Questions What do you think the main focus of the work with John should be to uphold the ethical principles of beneficence and non-maleficence?

Do you believe that a psychoeducational/relational model might be helpful?

Given John's deep depression, lack of motivation, and low energy, how would you, as his counsellor, plan to look after yourself in this work?

Rigid Thinking

Many survivors of religious abuse struggle with rigid thinking, which makes sense when repressed critical thinking, as visualised in Winell's chart of childhood religious indoctrination (no date), in the developmental years, is taken into consideration. Miller (2023, p. 31) categorises the effects into three categories. The first is 'impaired critical thinking', which manifests as 'difficulty determining fact from opinion, quickly dismissing nuance and difficulty compromising', while the second is recognised as 'binary thinking', which is 'categorizing things into extremes (good vs. bad), moralizing, and judging neutral ideas or actions as right or wrong'. The third category is 'false certainty', which Miller (2023, p. 31) describes as 'inflated confidence in the correctness of one's own stance, intolerance, poor listening skills, frequent confrontations, limited empathy, refusal to accept contracting evidence'. A client may, therefore, present in the therapeutic space with all of these forms of rigid thinking.

The dominant dualistic atmospheres that dominate fundamentalist groups mean that religious trauma survivors can be susceptible to 'a higher prevalence of psychosis or be vulnerable to a psychotic level of thinking' (Friedson, 2015, p. 705). Similarly, because of the high demands, expectations and perfectionism that are also present, 'it is possible that there may be a higher prevalence of obsessive and obsessive–compulsive difficulties among members of Fundamentalist religions' (Friedson, 2015, p. 705).

Case Study 6: Moira

Forty-year-old Moira is a returning client. The original sessions focused on the client's high levels of anxiety and obsessive–compulsive disorder (OCD) behaviours, which had started when she was eight. As a child, she was terrified of stepping on pavement lines and avoided them whenever possible.

CBT was used to help Moira understand her negative automatic thoughts as well as her unhelpful thinking habits in her first therapy. She quickly learned to rationalise her predictive and catastrophic thinking, and found that keeping thought diaries helped her to notice unhelpful thought patterns and challenge them. When the counselling sessions ended, she was in a better place with her anxiety levels and OCD behaviours more manageable. She was optimistic about her life going forward.

Moira recently returned for some further counselling. At the assessment, she stated that she had found counselling very helpful last time, but was again experiencing high levels of anxiety. She had also noticed increased compulsions and obsessions. However, the focus of fear this time was her faith, and she was seriously doubting whether she was a Christian at all. She was terrified that even a small 'sin' would send her to hell, for eternity. She described experiencing compulsive obsessions around buying only ethical products, the amount of coffee she drank, and the overwhelming compulsion to help every homeless person she saw. She believed that her sessions would only be helpful if there was prayer at the beginning of each one.

Reflective Questions Are any of the forms of rigid thinking, i.e. impaired critical thinking, binary thinking, and/or false certainty, evident in Moira's presentation?

Might cognitive behavioural thinking be a helpful way of working with this client again, or might an alternative theoretical modality be considered? If so, consider which theoretical approach might be helpful.

How might you respond to Moira in her expressed need for prayer at the start of a session for it to be successful?

Spiritual Bypassing

Spiritual bypassing refers:

> … to people leaning into spiritual or religious teachings as a primary method for addressing life distress and avoiding or 'bypassing' the mental and emotional work that might need to happen. The term has progressively come into wider use across religious and spiritual traditions. (Marich, 2024, p. 4)

Miller (2023, p. 111) suggests that there are two categories: admonishments and placations that are typically:

> … shame-based or suppression-based, and use judgment, invalidation or minimisation. They often bully members into silence or encourage them to blame themselves for negative experiences.

Examples of admonishments like 'God must be trying to teach you something' and placations such as 'everything happens for a reason' (Miller, 2023, pp. 111–112) are given, as well as an inventory that provides the opportunity for those who have been in a religious group to check whether they have been impacted by this. Religious trauma clients may use spiritual bypassing generally and in the therapeutic space. What is more, they may be distressed by what they perceive as their lack of ability to forgive those who have betrayed their trust. However, Marich (2024, p. 9) asserts that:

> … the forgiveness theology is the ultimate spiritual bypass – that is, using spiritual or religious concepts to practice avoidance of real human emotions and experiences.

She goes on to state that having the mindset of 'the past is the past, let's move on for the sake of healing bypasses will always prevent real change from happening in our systems and our world' (Marich, 2024, p. 10).

Case Study 7: Sophie

Sophie is in her late thirties and was referred for counselling by her minister. She grew up in a fundamentalist religious church, has a strong

Christian faith, and is one of the leaders. At the initial consultation, she explained that she had been referred for counselling because her fifteen-year marriage had ended. A few months previously, her husband had walked out and was living with a twenty-year-old with whom he had had an affair for the previous eighteen months.

Sophie is a strong believer in the sanctity of marriage and is devastated by recent events, as she had thought they would stay married 'until death do us part'. Although very tearful, she uses spiritual bypassing all the time to cope. Verses of scripture and placations such as 'I'll never be given more than I can handle' and 'everything happens for a reason' are thrown frequently into the room. She uses admonishments such as 'the Lord sees everything' and 'love the sinner and hate the sin' when speaking about her husband's behaviour. It is clear that she is very angry but uses it as a protective defence. The pace of the sessions is quick, and it is difficult to get a word in edgeways or connect with the client.

Reflective Questions If Sophie were your client, how might you deal with her constant use of spiritual bypassing?

How might you handle the potentially triggering effects for you, given the challenges of your strict religious upbringing?

Do you think that you would be able to connect with Sophie and build a therapeutic bond?

Grief and Loss

A client may present for therapy in deep grief. They may have left a high-demand religious group and lost family members, friends, and religious community as a result. Shunned and ostracised, they may also have lost their certainty of beliefs. A myriad of claims are made regarding the detrimental impact of being ostracised, for example, 'it unleashes a variety of physiological, affective, cognitive and behavioural responses' (Williams & Nida, 2011, p. 71), with identified common consequences being anxiety, panic, anger, guilt, depression, suicidal ideation, and tragically sometimes suicide completion (Zieman, 2018). Grief effects include sadness but can detrimentally affect the whole person with common symptoms such as headaches, chest pains, sleeplessness, and irrepressible crying (Selbie, 2024). The therapeutic space can be a safe space for a grieving client seeking to process loss and grief without judgement but with empathy and unconditional positive regard.

It is important to understand that exiting a group does not necessarily mean leaving a religion, although deconstructing, leaving, and reconstructing their belief system could accompany the grief journey. Zieman (2018) provides valuable psychoeducational information about shunning and also lists a plethora of techniques and survival strategies for those affected, for example, tips on downregulating the circuit of the nervous system, including reactivation of the ventral vagus nerve (Porges, 2017). Other helpful strategies include visualisation, coping techniques, and ways of managing unhelpful and racing thoughts, while tools of the faith, such as meditation and prayer, could be 'reframed as grounding methods' (Mayo-Beube, 2016, p. 6) with breathing as a foundational practice (Pasquale, 2015, p. 8).

Reframing and Reclaiming Identity

For a young person growing up in a fundamentalist religious group, the normal development of their unique identity is repressed by religious indoctrination and the inherent power and control dynamics. This has been likened to a layer of tarmac overlaying the authentic personality so that a pseudo-cult personality develops in its place (Jenkinson, 2008). For the survivor of religious abuse presenting as an adult for therapy, they may have become compliant, passive, and appeasing echoists as a survival mechanism; they may be unable to critically evaluate and may appear naïve in the outside world. It is vastly important for those born into a fundamentalist religious group to reframe it, and for those who grew up in a strict environment to reclaim theirs. However, the emergence or re-emergence of a client's authentic identity can come at relational cost, as those around the client might not like or approve of the changes.

References

Aguado, J. F. (2018). How a dysfunctional family functions like a cult. *ICSA Today, 9*(3), 2–7.

American Psychological Association. (2011). *Children and trauma update for mental health professionals.* https://www.apa.org/pi/families/resources/children-trauma-update

Beck, A. (2020, February 11–12). *CBT for working with post traumatic disorder.* SDS seminars live webcast training course, London.

British Association for Counselling and Psychotherapy. (2018). *Ethical framework for the counselling professions.* BACP.

Cole, M. (2023). Psychological effects of Christian teachings about sin and hell. *Mental Health, Religion & Culture.* https://doi.org/10.1080/136746762023.2261412

Cooper, M. (2008). *Essential research findings in counselling and psychotherapy: The facts are friendly.* Sage.

Cranney, S., Leman, J., Fergus, T. A., & Rowatt, W. C. (2018). Hell anxiety scale. *PsychTESTS.* https://doi.org/10.1037/t72689-000

Drumsta, R. (2023). *What is religious scrupulosity OCD?* August 4, 2025. https://www.rebekahdrumsta.com/blog/what-is-religious-scrupulosity-ocd

Fisher, J. (2017). *Healing the fragmented selves of trauma survivors: Overcoming internal self-alienation.* Routledge.

Friedson, M. L. (2015). Psychotherapy and the fundamentalist client: The aims and challenges of treating Jehovah's Witnesses. *Journal of Religious Health, 54*, 693–712. https://doi.org/10.1007/s10943-014-9946-8

Jenkinson, G. (2008). An investigation into cult pseudo-personality: What is it and how does it form? *Cultic Studies Review, 7*(3), 199–224.

Jenkinson, G. (2013). Working with cult survivors. *Therapy Today, BACP,* 18–21.

Jenkinson, G. (2019a, March). Out in the world: Post-cult recovery. *Therapy Today,* pp. 23–26.

Jenkinson, G. (2019b). *Post-cult counselling workbook. A guide for your recovery and growth.* Hope Valley Counselling.

Jenkinson, G. (2023). *Walking free from the trauma of coercive*. Routledge.

Karris, M. G. (2023). *The diabolical trinity.* SacraSage Press.

Keller, K. (2016). *Development of a spiritual abuse questionnaire.* [PhD dissertation, Texas Woman's University, pp. 129–130].

Knapp, P. J. (2021). *Understanding religious abuse and recovery. Discovering essential principles for hope and healing.* Pickwick.

Koch, D., & Edstrom, L. (2024). Development of the Spiritual Harm and Abuse Scale. *Journal for the Scientific Study of Religion, 61*(2), 476–506. https://doi.org/10.1111/jssr.12792

Marich, J. (2024). *You lied to me about God.* North Atlantic Books.

Mayo-Beube, M. (2016). *Recognising spiritual abuse in the context of the counselling professions.* BACP.

McBeath, A., & Greenles, P. (2016). Psychological and therapeutic issues associated with membership of high-demand religious groups. *Psychotherapy Section Review, 58*, 71–76.

Miller, A. C. (2023). *Religious trauma survival guide. Education and recovery tools for survivors and professionals.* Empathy Paradigm.

National Institute for Health Research. (2021). www.nihr.ac.uk

Novšak, R., Mandelj, T. R., & Simonič, B. (2012). Therapeutic implications of religious-related emotional abuse. *Journal of Aggression, Maltreatment and Trauma, 21*, 31–44. https://doi.org/10.1080/10926771.2011.627914

Pasquale, T. B. (2015). *Sacred wounds. A path to healing from spiritual trauma.* Chalice Press.

Porges, S. W. (2017). *The pocket guide to the polyvagal theory: The transformative power of feeling safe*. Norton.

Rothschild, B. with Rand, M. (2006). *Help for the helper:* The psychophysiology of compassion fatigue and vicarious trauma. W. W. Norton.

Roudkovski, K. (2024). *Understanding spiritual abuse. What it is and how to respond.* B&H Academic.

Sanderson, C. (2013). *Counselling skills for working with trauma.* Jessica Kingsley.

Selbie, J. (2024). *Divorcing religion. A memoir and survival handbook.* Prominence.

Snyder, K. (2023). *Shimmering around the edges. A memoir of OCD, reality, and finding God in uncertainty.* https://www.kathrinesnyder.com

Swindle, P. J. (2017). *A twisting of the sacred: The lived experience of religious abuse.* PhD thesis, University of North Carolina. https://www.proquest.com/openview/2f8757f55d11975590c5affc36b72169/1?pq-origsite=gscholar&cbl=18750

Swindle, P, J., Cashwell, C., & Tangen, J. L. (2024). *Counseling survivors of religious abuse.* Routledge.

Van der Kolk, B. (2014). *The body keeps the score.* Penguin Random House.

Weller, F. (2015). *The wild edge of sorrow. Rituals of renewal and the sacred work of grief*. North Atlantic Books.

Williams, K. D., & Nida, S. A. (2011). Ostracism: Consequences and coping. *Current Directions in Psychological Science, 20*(2), 71–75. https://doi.org/10.1177/0963721411402480

Zieman, B. (2017). *Cracking the cult code for therapists.* CreateSpace Independent Publishing Platform.

Zieman, B. (2018). *Shunned: A survival guide.* Amazon.

12

Concluding Thoughts

A Summary of the Beneficial and Challenging Effects of a Fundamentalist Religious Upbringing

There has never been a more pertinent time for counsellors, psychotherapists, and other practitioners to understand the benefits and challenges of a fundamentalist religious upbringing and the potential impact on adult health. Increasingly, those who have suffered spiritual abuse as children, young people, and adults are speaking out alongside high-profile cases attracting media attention, resulting in increasing public awareness. It is evident in the research findings that not all religious influences during the growing-up years are negative: bonding and belonging can be found, knowledge about religious matters can be gained, and religious practices can facilitate resilience.

Most of the extant literature focuses on the challenging, traumatic aspects of a strict religious upbringing. Kinmond et al., (2019, p. 1) recognise that child abuse linked to faith and belief (CALFB) is 'not a recent phenomenon, nor specific to any culture or faith', although it is often associated with satanic ritual abuse, witchcraft, and medical

G. Harvey, *Fundamentalist Religious Childhoods and Adult Mental Health and Wellbeing*, https://doi.org/10.1007/978-3-032-20140-9_12

neglect, mainly within Christianity. Religious abuse is far broader than those specific forms and happens in all religions. Traumatic experiences, especially those suffered in the formative years involving betrayal by the very people who should have been trustworthy, leave an imprinted legacy on victims, who may, after much healing, still suffer symptoms suggestive of complex post-traumatic stress disorder (C-PTSD) 'flare-ups' (Anderson, 2023, p. 206). Each person's understanding of their lived experiences is unique, and as explored in Chapter 8, they can detrimentally impact the six areas of functioning.

As depicted in Table 9.1, the co-researchers' religious statuses at the time of interview demonstrate that some survivors will reject all forms of religion, while others go through an evolution of beliefs from the ones that they grew up in. Some regard themselves as spiritual rather than religious, while the remaining participants express an openness to exploring spirituality at some point. McChesney (2025)*argues that the soul (as well as the body) keeps the score, and this aligns with* McConnaughey's (2022)*perspective that spiritual practices such as meditation, prayer, fasting, and study can be triggering for those traumatised by religion. She argues that although victims may often regard themselves as spiritual failures, the struggle with these practices is a trauma response rather than spiritual inadequacy.* This is an important understanding for therapists and spiritual directors alike, with McChesney (2025, p. 87) positing that some of the spiritual exercises used in spiritual direction, such as those of St. Ignatius, are helpful to healing 'spiritual injury'. *Yet, a religious trauma client might struggle to bond with any practitioner trying to help them because of the relational nature of religious abuse.*

Responding Appropriately to Disclosures

The findings of one survey-based study with counsellor participants, which was thematically analysed, emphasised the importance of responding effectively by listening and attending while protecting confidentiality (Kinmond et al., 2019). Oakley et al., (2024, p. 10) also stress the importance of 'responding well' and recognised that revealing spiritual abuse can be very distressing, with victims commonly fearing that they will not be believed. *All practitioners need to bear in mind the importance of safeguarding and respond appropriately to disclosures of religious abuse while being open to the possibility of the authorities needing to be informed.*

Boundary Setting and Self-Compassion

One of the biggest challenges for those healing from religious abuse can be setting boundaries to allow themselves not to be taken for granted. In a high-demand religious group, these are frequently blurred and violated. The setting of boundaries can consequently be an alien concept for survivors, but the practitioner can model the importance of them in the therapeutic work. *The client might be helped by the counsellor disclosing if they themselves have suffered spiritual abuse, because this might indicate some understanding; however, the sharing of the professional's experience would need to be kept minimal.*

Many victims are filled with shame, which is 'the demoralising belief that we are broken or fundamentally inadequate' (Miller, 2023, p. 120). The antidote to this is self-compassion, which is also likely to be an alien concept for those who have experienced religious abuse. Miller (2023, pp. 120–21) suggests starting to address it by noticing the internal dialogue and 'replacing it with a more empowering and compassionate alternative' and helpfully provides a comparison table. For example, shame's message is that 'I am defective/broken' while self-compassion says, 'I've been hurt but not broken'.

Practitioners' Awareness of Their Own Biases and Cultural Backgrounds

The counsellor participants in Kinmond et al's. (2019) research showed evidence of assumptions being made about religious communities where CALFB is likely to occur, with the recommendation being made that counsellors need to be aware of their own cultural background, prejudices, and assumptions, and what impact they may have on client work of this nature because both trauma and healing are subjective (Anderson, 2023). Friedson (2015, p. 711)*argues for 'culturally sensitive psychotherapeutic interventions' for current and ex-JWs and other clients distressed because of their fundamentalist religious encounters.*

Vicarious Trauma and Practitioner Self-Care

The guidelines of the British Association for Counselling and Psychotherapy (BACP, 2018) include the ethical principle of self-respect and encourage practitioner self-care. *When working with survivors of religious abuse, therapists must be aware of the dangers of vicarious trauma.* This has been defined as 'the negative transformation in the self of the helper that comes about as a result of empathic engagement with survivors' trauma material and a sense of responsibility or commitment to help' (McCann and Pearlman, 1990, cited in Sanderson, 2013, p. 280). A counsellor can suffer vicarious trauma when clients describe graphic scenes of abuse, especially if the professional has also been abused. While empathy is a great asset, it has consequences because 'even when a therapist was not actually involved in the client's trauma, she can vicariously experience it in her nervous system' (Rothschild, 2006, p. 15). It is clear that to provide a good standard of care, resilience is required, which is 'the capacity to work with the client's concerns without being personally diminished' (BACP Ethical Framework, 2018, p. 4). *Some of the factors that facilitate this include being mindfully grounded in sessions, maintaining a healthy work/life balance and a good support network, adherence to compassionate self-care, not taking on too many trauma clients, and utilising supervision to its maximum.*

Training and Supervision

While there is now some recognition of the importance of religion and spirituality within the counselling profession (Miller, 1999), the influence of childhood religion on developmental and later wellbeing is often overlooked (Hansen, 1998), and this is of great concern. Although the introduction of 'The Churchill Framework' (Churchill, 2021) provides guidelines for working with religion and spirituality in the therapeutic space, it may be limited in its application to religions beyond Christianity, plus some counsellors still feel ill-equipped to work with such matters and need further training (Christodoulidi, 2011; Hofmann & Walach, 2011). Hunt's (2024, p. 1601) three-part survey-based research identified 'the absence of training on religion/spirituality in the therapeutic curriculum' with trainees wanting study programmes to be more affirming of their religious or spiritual beliefs and the impact of those on clinical practice. Kinmond et al. and's (2019, p. 664) findings also identified the need for training for counsellors, stating that they needed to be 'better equipped' to work with CALFB.

The importance of appropriate, informed supervision being available for counsellors working with these matters was emphasised by Gubi and Jacobs (2009), with Kinmond et al. (2019) emphasising the need for more research and direction for those working with CALFB issues. *Having rigorous assessment processes in place is also vital* (Cashwell & Swindle, 2018, p. 182)*so that counsellors and psychotherapists can be supported to work ethically, within their levels of competency (BACP, 2018),* and with the knowledge that such stories can contain healthy connection and/or manipulative, powerful control, as 'both sides of the coin' may have been present in the client's childhood.

While there has been a burgeoning interest in religion and health within recent years, most research on this topic has been carried out in the USA, with Oakley and Kinmond's (2013) work on spiritual abuse being groundbreaking in the UK. This and other collaborative work by these authors focuses on occurrences within Christian churches, and it is of note that debate exists as to whether spiritual abuse is a category in its own right. This is the perspective of the Evangelical Alliance, an influential UK evangelical Christian organisation, which argues that spiritual abuse is a faulty concept because, unlike other forms of abuse, it is not covered by the legal structures in this country, whereas if it were legalised, the sincerely held beliefs and systems of conservative churches might be victimised (Parsons, 2018). Godina's (2014) qualitative research to inform the UK social work profession, involving only Seventh-day

Adventist participants, also has a narrow focus on a particular group within Christianity.

This qualitative research study matters because it has uniquely focused on the stories of counsellors in the UK regarding the influence of fundamentalist religious upbringing on mental health and wellbeing in adulthood, and it makes an original contribution to knowledge in this regard. While the literature review demonstrated that there is an over-abundance of texts on religion and health and religious fundamentalism generally, many of them of US origin, the research gap that exists is around the effects on mental health and wellbeing in later life for those born and/or raised within strict religious settings within the UK. While one piece of research is unable to fill the gap, this project has aimed to partially meet the lack of UK literature on this topic.

Future Research

In parallel with the findings of the literature review, which shows that most researchers have used Western Christian participants, this imbalance is also true for this study. The researcher is a white woman looking through a much-evolved but still Christian faith lens, so this bias has been unintentionally perpetuated. There were single-voice representations from Islam and Judaism. *Future research needs to include a greater number of participants who have experienced a Muslim or Jewish upbringing or who have worked with clients with those strict religious childhoods; otherwise, more research just contributes to the literature bias.*

It is the author's conviction that research on growing up within other religions, Hinduism, for example, and others, such as Roman Catholicism or minority religions, such as the Quakers, and the impact on mental health and wellbeing in adulthood, would significantly contribute to understanding around this important subject, as would contributions from a larger number of participants. All of this could make possible a greater recognition of the importance of such stories at the macro-level of society, as well as the micro-level of interactions between clients and therapists, ministers, rabbis, imams, and their followers, and spiritual directors and their directees, so that people with such experiences, both positive and negative, seeking help can be ethically and knowledgeably supported.

The Current Religious Context

Religion is still an integral part of contemporary life for some, with a continuum existing from liberal at one end to ultra-ultra strict at the other end in all religions. Singer (2024, p. 62) urges churches to become more 'trauma-informed' so that they can prevent and respond appropriately to abuse and minister to those who have been harmed, and this needs to be made a priority in all religious communities.

This is pertinent at this time because there is 'a marked attitudinal shift', increased acceptance, and openness in how friends talk about religion than in previous generations (Ash, 2025, p. 16). She states that in the more liberal Christian denominations, church attendance is continuing to drop, compared with more conservative religious communities, where attendance continues to grow. If this assertion is true, then there is no better time than now for all religious communities to become trauma-informed, for researchers to carry out ethical research, and for practitioners to be psycho-educated on the benefits and challenges of a fundamentalist religious upbringing. After all, Pasquale (2015, p. 3) states:

> … what I found is that no religion is immune to fundamentalism. Religion is made up of humans, and our humanity can be the best of us or get the best of us.

References

Anderson, L. E. (2023). *When religion hurts you*. Brazos Press.

Ash, L. (2025). *Don't forget we're here forever. A new generation's search for religion*. Bloomsbury Circus.

British Association for Counselling & Psychotherapy (2018). Ethical framework for the counselling professions. Lutterworth: BACP.

Cashwell, C. S., & Swindle, P. J. (2018). When religion hurts: Supervising cases of religious abuse. *The Clinical Supervisor, 37*(1), 182–203. https://doi.org/10.1080/07325223.2018.1443305

Christodoulidi, F. (2011). Counselling, spirituality, and culture. In W. West (Ed.), *Exploring therapy, spirituality and healing.* Palgrave Macmillan.

Churchill, H. (2021). The Churchill Framework: A core-competence framework when working with clients' religious/spiritual issues in clinical practice. *Accord, 110*(Spring), 21–27.

Friedson, M. L. (2015). Psychotherapy and the fundamentalist client: The aims and challenges of treating Jehovah's Witnesses. *Journal of Religious Health, 54*, 693–712. https://doi.org/10.1007/s10943-014-9946-8

Godina, L. (2014). Religion and parenting: Ignored relationship? *Child and Family Social Work, 19*, 381–390. https://doi.org/10.1111/cfs.12054

Gubi, P. M., & Jacobs, R. (2009). Exploring the impact on counsellors of working with spiritually abused clients. *Mental Health, Religion & Culture, 12*, 191–204. https://doi.org/10.1080/13674670802441509

Hansen, C. (1998). Long-term effects of religious upbringing. *Mental Health, Religion & Culture, 1*(2), 91–111. 1080/13674679808406502

Hofmann, L., & Walach, H. (2011). Spirituality and religiosity in psychotherapy—A representative survey among German psychotherapists. *Psychotherapy Research, 21*(2), 179–192.

Hunt, J. (2024). Religion and spirituality in therapeutic training in the UK: A survey of current and recent trainees. *Counselling and Psychotherapy Research, 24*, 1600–1611. https://doi.org/10.1002/capr.12807

Kinmond, K., Oakley, L., Humphreys, J., & Dioum, M. (2019). Child abuse linked to faith or belief: An important issue for counselling practice. *British Journal of Guidance & Counselling, 47*(6), 659–668. https://doi.org/10.1080/03069885.2017.1370696

McChesney, R. W. (2025). *The soul also keeps the score*. Liturgical Press.

McConnaughey, J. (2022). *Trauma in the pews*. Berry Powell Press.

Miller, A. C. (2023). *Religious trauma survival guide. Education and recovery tools for survivors and professionals.* Empathy Paradigm.

Miller, G. A. (1999). The development of the spiritual focus in counselling and counsellor education. *Journal of Counselling & Development, 77*, 498–501. https://doi.org/10.1002/j.1556-6676.1999.tb02478.x

Oakley, L., & Kinmond, K. (2013). *Breaking the silence on spiritual abuse*. Palgrave MacMillan.

Oakley, L., Kinmond, K., & Blundell, P. (2024). Responding well to spiritual abuse: Practice implications for counselling and psychotherapy. *British Journal of Guidance and Counselling, 52*(2), 189–206. https://doi.org/10.1080/03069885.2023.2283883

Parsons, S. (2018). *Surviving church. Exploring abuse in the church. Why does it happen? How can we move on?* http://survivingchurch.org//2018/02/06/evangelical-alliance-on-spiritual-abuse-unhelpful-and-confusing

Pasquale, T. B. (2015). *Sacred wounds*. Chalice Press.

Rothschild, B. with Rand, M. (2006), Help for the helper: The psychophysiology of compassion fatigue and vicarious trauma. W. W. Norton.

Sanderson, C. (2013), Counselling Skills for Working with Trauma. London: Jessica Kingsley Publishers.

Singer, P. (2024). Towards a more trauma-informed church: Equipping faith communities to prevent and respond to abuse. *Currents in Theology and Mission, 51*(1), 62–76.

Index

G. Harvey, *Fundamentalist Religious Childhoods and Adult Mental Health and Wellbeing*, https://doi.org/10.1007/978-3-032-20140-9

The manufacturer's authorised representative in the EU is Springer Nature Customer Service Centre GmbH, Europaplatz 3, 69115 Heidelberg, Germany. If you have any concerns regarding our products, please contact ProductSafety@springernature.com

Printed and bound by CPI Group (UK) Ltd, Croydon, CR0 4YY

17/09/2026

02218454-0006